APHRODISI

Belate
March 1987
It should be fun finding
out if they _work_

have

Chris, Ann,
    Sarah & Peto.

APHRODISIACS
FACT AND FICTION

Peter Levene

JAVELIN BOOKS
POOLE · DORSET

First published in the UK 1985 by Javelin Books,
Link House, West Street, Poole, Dorset BH15 1LL

Copyright © 1985 Peter Levene

Distributed in the United States by
Sterling Publishing Co., Inc.,
2 Park Avenue, New York, N.Y. 10016.

British Library Cataloguing in Publication Data

Levene, Peter
  Aphrodisiacs : fact and fiction.
  1. Cookery   2. Aphrodisiacs
  I. Title
  641.5   TX840.A/

ISBN 0 7137 1568 5

*Typeset by Colset Pte. Ltd., Singapore
Printed in Great Britain by Hazell, Watson and Viney, Aylesbury*

Contents

PART I –
THE APHRODISIACS

1 Introduction

What is an 'aphrodisiac'? The dictionary definition is 'a drug or food which stimulates sexual desire'. It may be self-administered or, as in the case of the olden-day love potions, given unbeknown to the recipient. Are there such things, and do they work? Is the answer 'all in the mind'? These are the questions I shall try to find the answers to. I hope that you will enjoy accompanying me in this quest, and that ultimately you will benefit from it.

Aphrodisiacs fall into four main categories.

DRUGS

This group contains a variety of drugs, most of which have been known and used for centuries all over the world, and which for the most part are very dangerous if used repetitively or in any but the smallest quantities. One has to accept that there are drugs that can kill, can cause drowsiness or hallucinations, can sedate or stimulate, and even make one tell the truth. It is obvious then that there are drugs that can make you feel more sexy.

FOODS AND SPICES

Into this group come the various foods which have acquired a reputation over the years as aphrodisiacs. Nowadays, oysters, ginseng, curry, and foods with a high vitamin E content readily come to mind, but in the past other less likely foods have had the limelight, such as hot chocolate and potatoes. (More of these later.) As far as their effectiveness is concerned, if you believe and have faith all things are possible!

SYMBOLIC ITEMS

This group comprises items which have been used, usually for hundreds, sometimes for thousands, of years. They were originally chosen for their sexual origins or likenesses, and were usually eaten, although sometimes made into an ointment. I do not have any recipes for powdered rhinoceros horn, or dried placentas, or animal testicles, or dehydrated beetles, but this was the type of base for the love potions of the past. No doubt they worked if the recipient believed they would.

ODOURS

Natural odours are a means of attraction in flowers for insects to pollinate them, and, in mammals in their wild state, odour glands are used to attract a mate. It is possible that this still works to a degree in humans, but the use of perfumes to enhance the effect has been used throughout the ages.

The purpose of this book is to explore the history of aphrodisiacs, and to put forward some suggestions as to the genuineness of a few items. If, after reading Part I, you think there may be some truth in what you have read, then I dare you to carry the experiment further, and try some of the recipes in Part II.

Let us return to the name 'aphrodisiac' for a moment. This is not a new word — it was listed in the *Glossographia Anglicana Nova* of 1719, an early dictionary, as 'APHRODISIACKS, Things that excite Lust or Venery'. The name comes from the Greek goddess of love, Aphrodite, so perhaps we should start our quest by finding out more about this goddess, and why her name has been associated throughout the centuries with sexual desire.

2 Aphrodite

Aphrodite was the Greek goddess of erotic love and beauty, and was called Venus by the Romans. Her father was Uranus, the most ancient of the gods, and their first ruler. His children were the Titans, the Cyclopes, and the hundred-handed monsters with fifty heads — Cottus, Briareus, and Gyges. He hated the monsters and the Cyclopes, and threw them into Tartarus, which was a kind of hell, as far distant from the earth as the earth was from the sky, where they were kept in constant torment.

For revenge, their mother Ge encouraged the Titans to attack their father and overthrow him. They did so, led by the youngest son Cronus, who, armed with a flint sickle given to him by his mother, surprised Uranus while he was asleep, and grasping his father's genitals in his left hand castrated him with repeated cuts from the flint sickle, and then threw both the sickle and the genitals into the sea by Cape Drepanum.

From the droplets of Uranus's blood sprang the Three Erinnyes or Furies, who were of hideous aspect, and these avenged the perpetrators of crimes against the laws of society.

The Titans then released the Cyclopes and the hundred-handed monsters from Tartarus, and made Cronus the new ruler of the earth. As soon as he was in command, Cronus sent the Cyclopes and the monsters back to perpetual torment in Tartarus, and married his sister Rhea.

Meanwhile, from the foam which gathered in the sea around the genitals of Uranus, Aphrodite arose naked from the sea on a scallop shell, and sailed to take up residence in Paphos, in Cyprus, after finding the first island she landed on, Cythera, too small. These were her chief seats of worship — Cythera and

Cyprus. On her arrival in Paphos the daughters of Themis rushed to clothe her, and wherever she trod grass and flowers sprang from the earth. The dove, swan, swallow and the bird called Iynx drew her chariot, or served as her messengers; and these, together with the myrtle, rose, apple and poppy, were sacred to her.

She had a magic girdle that made anyone who saw it fall in love with its wearer, and although she was asked many times by the other goddesses to lend it to them she almost always refused, wishing to keep its love-inducing powers for herself. Zeus later gave her in marriage to Hephaestus, the unromantic lame god of fire, but she constantly deceived him with Ares, the god of war, and her first three children were all fathered by Ares. Hephaestus knew nothing of her infidelity until one night when she stayed too long in Ares' bed and was seen by Helius, who immediately ran to tell Hephaestus. Her husband was stunned and extremely angry, and hastened to his forge, where he hammered out a bronze hunting net as fine as gossamer, but unbreakable. He tied this to the posts and sides of his marriage bed, and when Aphrodite later returned he told her he had to go away for a short time to Lemnos, another island.

Aphrodite declined to go with him, and as soon as he was out of sight she sent for Ares, who hurried over and was soon in bed with her. When dawn arrived they found themselves entangled in the net, completely naked, and unable to escape. Later that morning Hephaestus returned and surprised them there, and summoned all the gods to come and ridicule them. He then announced that he would not release them until Zeus had repaid all the valuable marriage gifts Hephaestus had given to him. Zeus was disgusted and refused to hand back the gifts, saying that any vulgar disputes between a husband and wife had nothing to do with him.

Poseidon, who had instantly fallen in love with Aphrodite at

7

the sight of her naked body, undertook to make Ares repay the gifts if he were released, and in the event of Ares not repaying them he guaranteed to repay the debt himself, and to marry Aphrodite into the bargain. On these conditions Ares and Aphrodite were released. The gifts were never repaid, but Hephaestus did not seek a divorce because he was still madly in love with her.

Aphrodite returned to Paphos, and there, surprisingly for her, repulsed the passionate advances of Hermes. Zeus took pity on Hermes and sent an eagle to snatch Aphrodite's sandal as she bathed in the river, and carry it back to Hermes. In order to have it returned she had to submit to his desires, and the resultant child of his blackmail was Hermaphroditus, a dual-sexed being, whose name was made up from those of both his parents.

To show her gratitude to Poseidon she bore him two sons, Rhodus and Herophilus. Her next conquest was Dionysus, and she bore him Priapus who was an ugly child with huge genitals — wished on him by Hera, who disapproved of Aphrodite's promiscuity. Hera was Aphrodite's mother in law. Aphrodite had many more lovers among the gods, and Anchises and Adonis amongst the mortals.

She competed with Hera and Athena, for the prize of the golden apple, in a contest to find the most beautiful of the goddesses, and bribed the judge, Paris, with the hand of Helen, Queen of Sparta, who was the most beautiful mortal woman. As her bribe was better than those offered by her competitors, she was duly selected by Paris, who then abducted Helen. This started the Trojan War, in which Aphrodite sided with the Trojans and protected Paris as much as she was able. Hera sided with the Greeks, because Paris had chosen Aphrodite in preference to her. Paris was eventually mortally wounded after killing Achilles, but that is another story.

The Fates had assigned one divine duty only to Aphrodite, and that was to make love.

In works of art, she is often represented with her son Eros, whose father is unknown, but could have been Hermes, Ares, or even Zeus. Of the statues which remain of her, the most notable is the celebrated Venus de Milo in the Louvre, Paris, which was found in 1820 on the island of Milos. Other notable statues are Aphrodite of Capua, and the Medicean Aphrodite in Florence.

The concept the Greeks had of Aphrodite was undoubtedly based on the Phoenician goddess Astarte, who was brought in in the early days by Phoenician traders, or on Ishtar, who was the Assyrian and Babylonian equivalent of Astarte.

For reference purposes, the Roman counterparts of the Greek gods mentioned above are as follows:

Aphrodite — Venus	Zeus — Jupiter	Hephaestus — Vulcan
Ares — Mars	Poseidon — Neptune	Hermes — Mercury
Dionysus — Bacchus	Hera — Juno	Eros — Cupid

Just to round off the story, a bit of background knowledge about the rest of the characters will not come amiss for those who are interested. Cronus feared a prophecy that he in turn would be overthrown by one of his children, and in order to avert this disaster he swallowed each infant at birth. Rhea duped Cronus by bearing Zeus secretly in a cave, and wrapping a stone in swaddling clothes and giving that to Cronus to swallow instead. After he had grown up, Zeus tricked his father into drinking an emetic. Cronus then vomited up his other children, Hades, Poseidon and Hera. The three brothers, Zeus, Hades and Poseidon, then overthrew Cronus and the Titans and divided the universe between them. Hades received the underworld, Poseidon the ocean, and Zeus the sky. Although all three had equal rights to the earth, Zeus was acknowledged chief of the gods.

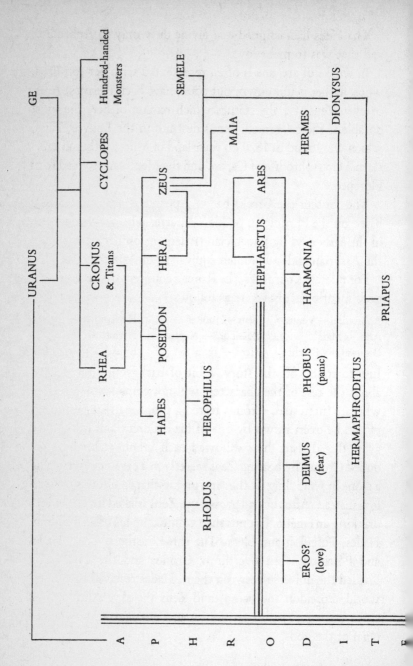

10

3 Customs World-wide

Aphrodisiacs have a long and fascinating history. Looking back we find that the ancient Hebrews used caper berries (*Capparis spinosa*) for sexual stimulation, and in India in the sixth century BC one of the medical authorities recommended the eating of animal testicles as a cure for impotence. This form of aphrodisiac has been used universally through the ages, for obvious reasons. Perhaps one of the most well-known aphrodisiacs is powdered rhinoceros horn. The rhinoceros has been hunted down since the Middle Ages solely for the plunder of its horn, and because of this is now an endangered species. We can see why when we learn that the horn is worth about half its weight in gold on the Oriental market. The use of love potions sometimes had a very serious outcome. Aristotle (384–322 BC), the famous Greek philosopher, once wrote of a woman who was brought before the judges for poisoning her husband. She pleaded not guilty, saying that she only wished to revive his dying love. She was acquitted. This form of defence is not recommended nowadays.

In the ancient world great claims were made for alcohol, opium, hashish etc.; Xenocrates (Greek philosopher 369–314 BC) said that the sap of mallows excited the sexual passion of women. Theophrastus, another Greek philosopher (327–287 BC), described the effect of holding a certain plant in his hand which had enabled a man to achieve sexual relations seventy times in one night. He forgot to name the plant, unfortunately. Roman women were admonished by Juvenal, the Roman poet, in the first century for dosing their husbands with love potions which only caused premature senility, dizziness and loss of memory. Rumour has it that another Roman poet, Lucretius

(99–55 BC) went mad and committed suicide after having such a potion. Pliny, in the first century AD, spoke of a famous aphrodisiac called thelygonon, which was a plant whose seeds were said to resemble testicles. He also urged that men anxious about their virility should eat the testicles of a horse.

In ancient civilisations the use of a placenta played a large part. In fact they have been used by different peoples up to modern times, and were usually thought to ensure undying love if a lover was made to eat it unknowingly. A Chinese physician, Tung P'in, in the twelfth century, recommended cooking the placenta in alcohol, kneading it, and then serving it as dumplings with various herbs and powders. In medieval China, the favourite solution of the court physicians for lost potency was the consumption of fresh human brains.

Looking around the rest of the world we learn that the men of the Arunta tribe in Australia fed their women kangaroo testicles to stimulate their desire. Some American Indians, not being blessed with having kangaroos handy, made do with the testicles of beavers as the main ingredients of love philtres.

In India if a girl wished to attract a man sexually, she would prepare betel nuts or tobacco, and hide it in his pouch. The Creoles of Louisiana, when preparing a love philtre, roasted the hearts of hummingbirds, then ground them into a powder, and sprinkled this powder over the object of their desires.

In Nova Scotia the intended was given a drink of water in which the plant Spiranthes had been steeped. One recipe obtained from an American Negro was to 'place a live frog in an anthill until all that is left is its bones. Then keep the heart-shaped bone yourself, but hook the hook-shaped bone onto the clothing of your beloved.'

In Indonesia a girl would hide her girdle in the clothing of the one she loved. In Newfoundland an apple would be pricked full of holes, then carried under the left arm for a while, before giving it to the beloved. The Southern Slavs used to wear the entire body of a bat as an amulet to arouse sexual desire in their beloved. In Hungary the girls used to rub their blood onto their beloved's hair.

During the nineteenth century a wide range of aphrodisiacs were being manufactured in various countries. A typical example was in Cincinatti, in 1858, where Dr William A. Raphael claimed that his 'Cordial Invigorant' at three dollars a bottle could make possible 'the wonderful prolongation of the attributes of manhood'.

Nowadays, psychologists tend to think that impotence is caused more by the mind than the body. In past ages, however, it was thought to have been caused by witchcraft, and even provided grounds for divorce if sorcery could be proved. The ninth-century philosopher, Costa ben Luca, cured a certain great noble of his time from being bewitched and made impotent by prescribing an ancient aphrodisiac of crow's gall and sesame ointment. The great noble believed in the cure, and was relieved of his imaginary complaint. Other remedies have included ant salve, raven's bile in oil, and smoke from a dead man's tooth.

In England spell books or Grimoires were written somewhere between the sixteenth and eighteenth centuries, and they included spells from much earlier times. They contained recipes for all manner of things, including the following.

'To Make A Girl Dance Naked — write on virgin parchment a certain character with the blood of a bat. Cut it on a stone over which a Mass has been said, and place it beneath the door sill through which the girl will walk. Having walked over it she will undress and dance naked continually until she dies, unless the character is removed first.'

'A Love Charm — if a woman is frigid, take the members of a wolf, and burn them together with the hairs from his cheeks and eyebrows, and give them to her to drink unknowingly. She will become passionate and desire no other man.'

Love philtres were in great demand in Medieval Britain, and often had an aphrodisiac base. Herbs, powdered rhinoceros horn, and most new foods brought back from sea voyages and explorations were assumed to provoke lust.

In the North of England they used to have a love charm peculiar to St Faith's Day, 6th October. It went like this: 'A flour-cake is made (the ingredients being flour, spring-water, salt, and sugar) by three maidens or three widows, each taking an equal part. It is baked before the fire in an oven, no one speaking during the process, and each must turn it three times. It is divided, when ready, into three equal parts; each cuts her share into nine small slices, and passes each slice three times through a wedding-ring, the property of some woman who has been married not less than seven years. Then they undress, and during the time they are so occupied, they must eat the slices repeating these lines:

> O good St Faith, be kind tonight,
> And bring to me my heart's delight:
> Let me my future husband view,
> And be my visions chaste and true.

They all sleep in one bed, and the ring must be placed at the head of it; and then they are sure to obtain the desired object.'

In 1563 a man was reported to have cured his impotence with an ointment comprised of the bile of a raven, in oil. In 1676 J. H. Moliter, a professor of philosophy and medicine, advised anyone who had become the victim of a love philtre to take a mineral bath containing alum, antimony, arsenic, nitre, salt, sulphur and vitriol, and stated that this was an infallible cure.

J. Hartman, professor of chemistry at the University of Marburg in the seventeenth century, advised emetics, holy water and antimony taken internally. In 1689 there was a reference to ants being used in an aphrodisiac ointment. In the seventeenth century hot chocolate was considered an aphrodisiac.

In 1723, an unknown author, on his return from Ireland, wrote that the Irish were very partial to love philtres. One method was as follows: 'The Spark that's resolved to sacrifice his youth and vigour on a Damsel, whose coyness will not accept of his Love-Oblations, he threads a Needle with the Hair of her Head, and then running it thro' the most fleshy part of a dead Man, as the brawn of the Arms, Thigh, or the Calf of the Leg, the Charm has that virtue in it, as to make her run mad for him whom she so lately slighted.'

In the twentieth century a whole host of medicines and tablets appeared on the market containing different variations of iron carbonate, calcium carbonate, dandelions, strychnine, testosterone, yohimbine and various vitamins. Dr Theodore Hendrik van de Vende (1873–1937) held that yohimbine is a genuine aphrodisiac, but much too dangerous for general usage. He also recommended meat, particularly venison, and stated that eggs are also a sexual stimulant. Slightly behind these, he recommended beets, carrots, turnips, celery, artichokes, asparagus and crayfish soup.

Throughout history two names have continually been associated with aphrodisiacs — cantharides and mandrake or mandragora.

4 Cantharides and Mandrake

Cantharides (Spanish Flies) was mentioned by Aristotle as being an aphrodisiac, and he also advised oil of peppermint for the same use. Cantharadin is contained in the dried bodies of the blister beetle, and in the bodies of other beetles of the same family. Doctors and priests in olden times used to suffocate the beetle in hot vinegar fumes, then dry them and powder their bodies. If any but the smallest amount of cantharides is swallowed, a destructive reaction occurs in all the mucus membranes of the body such as the throat, stomach, mouth and intestines. It can also damage other organs, such as the kidneys. During this time a state of licentiousness may occur, and this is probably whence the reputation of an aphrodisiac arose. A too-large dose can cause death in 16–24 hours from asphyxia after excruciating pain.

It has always been known to be dangerous, from ancient times until the present day, but throughout the ages has been used as an aphrodisiac regardless. In the Middle Ages it was widely used in love potions. At the beginning of this century there were several officinal preparations in the forms of ointments, plasters etc. available, and a tincture of cantharides for internal use. It was used as a counter-irritant in neuralgia, or to relieve congestion in pleurisy, pericarditis, meningitis etc. The tincture was occasionally used in medicinal doses for skin diseases, enuresis in children, and as a diuretic.

Mandrake is native to southern Europe, and is a member of the potato family. It has been used as an aphrodisiac for thousands of years. It has always been thought to cure sterility and promote passion, and was used as an anaesthetic as well as an aphrodisiac. It contains atropine and scopolamine and can cause vomiting, mental confusion and death if taken in large enough quantities.

The mandrake is mentioned in *Genesis* 30 (14–16), when, referring to her barrenness, Rachel said: 'Leah, Give me, I pray thee, of thy son's mandrakes.' And they worked! The Hebrews called the yellow fruits 'Love Apples'.

The ancient Greeks used it as an anaesthetic in surgical operations, and it was used as such well into the Middle Ages. To obtain aphrodisiacal effects the root was steeped in wine or vinegar, and its erotic properties were so well known that Aphrodite was sometimes called Mandragoris. In the fourth century BC Theophrates recommended that the root be scraped and soaked in vinegar, as an aphrodisiac and a cure for sleeplessness. He stated that the plant should only be gathered after drawing three circles about it with a sword whilst facing west, whilst an assistant danced round in a circle chanting magic prayers. Pliny agreed with this, and added that it should not be gathered with the wind blowing directly into your face because of the stink!

Theophrastus (about 230 BC), who wrote the first Greek *History of Plants*, referred to it: 'The leaf mixed with meal is useful for wounds, and the root for erysipelas (acute inflammation of the lymphatic vessels of the skin, caused by streptococcal infection). When scraped and steeped in vinegar, it is also used for gout, for sleeplessness, and for love potions. It is administered in wine or vinegar.'

Dioscorides, the Greek physician in the first century AD, also spoke of mandrake as an aphrodisiac, and said in addition that mandragora wine should be used as a surgical anaesthetic. This wine was sometimes given to those about to be hung or crucified.

In some parts of Greece, young men still carry bits of mandrake root as love charms. In Arabia it was called the Devil's

Candle, because it shone at night. This phenomenon was caused by glow-worms, which thrive in the damp atmosphere of the leaves. In western Europe the root was even believed to cause conception if placed under the bed, and it was 'common knowledge' that elephants ate this plant to improve their sex life. Mandrake was supposed to flourish beneath the gallows, and to spring from the droplets of the executed corpses. Reminiscences of the birth of Aphrodite!

Mandrake is mentioned countless times in English literature, for example, John Donne (c. 1571–1631) wrote in *Go and Catch a Falling Star*: 'Get with child a Mandrake root'; and Shakespeare in *Othello*: 'Not poppy, nor mandragora, nor all the drowsy syrups of the world.' The shape of the mandrake root resembled the human form so much that in England they were differentiated by calling some *man*drakes, and others *woman*drakes. They were thought to shriek when plucked from the ground, and the noise of this shriek killed or sent mad anyone not blocking his ears against it. Shakespeare again, in *Romeo and Juliet*:

'And shrieks like mandrakes torn out of the earth,

That living mortals, hearing them, run mad.'

Human hands were not to come into contact with the plant's destructive properties, and it was believed the only way it could safely be uprooted was by moonlight, over appropriate prayer and ritual. The method for doing this was to attach a black dog to the plant by a cord, and throw a piece of bread for the dog to leap at. As the plant was pulled from the ground, the shriek was supposed to kill the dog instantly.

Because of the powers associated with the plant, its value rocketed, and a thriving counterfeit trade soon arose, and was carried on for several centuries. The counterfeit roots were usually bryony carved into human shape. Sometimes tiny cuts were made and wheat or grass seeds planted, so that when the shoots emerged they would resemble pubic hair.

Incidentally, witches were supposed to use the mandrake to make effigies of the person they intended to harm. Coles writes that witches 'take likewise the Roots of Mandrake, and make thereof an ugly Image, by which they represent the person on whom they intend to exercise their Witchcraft.' Bacon (1561–1626) wrote: 'Some plants there are, but rare, that have a mossy or downy root, and likewise that have a number of threads, like beards; as mandrakes, whereof Witches and Imposters make an ugly image, giving it the form of a face at the top of the root and leave those strings to make a broad beard down to the foot.' The remedy against this type of witchcraft was to put 'some of the bewitched person's water, with a quantity of pins, needles and nails, into a bottle, cork them up and set them before the fire, in order to confine the spirit: but this sometimes did not prove sufficient, as it would often force the cork out with a loud noise, like that of a pistol, and cast the contents of the bottle to a considerable height.'

The witch's bottle was very popular, and was usually partially filled with some of the victim's urine, hair or nail clippings, together with some other items such as pins, iron nails or thorns, and then firmly corked and boiled on the fire at midnight with all the doors and windows closed, and everyone sitting in silence. The witch was meant to suffer great pain all this while. If the cork were to pop out she would escape, and if the bottle exploded she would die. The most popular type of bottle was a bellarmine, called after Cardinal Robert Bellarmine (1542–1621). These were stoneware jugs imported from the Rhineland in the late sixteenth and seventeenth centuries, a number of which have been dug up by archaeologists. This method of breaking a witch's spell was employed into the late nineteenth century, when jam jars were used instead.

Incidentally, contrary to popular belief, hardly any witches were burnt in England. They were usually hanged after a trial by water. This consisted of being stripped naked and then immersed in a pond or river or such like, sometimes with their left thumb tied to their right toe, and their right thumb tied to their left toe. If they floated they were adjudged to have been repelled by the Waters of Baptism, and therefore guilty, and hanged. If they sank and were drowned, they were innocent. Another popular method was by finding private marks on their bodies. These were usually warts, moles or spots. Burning at the stake was the usual punishment on the continent and in Scotland. In Scotland alone well over 4,000 'witches' were burnt.

The travesty of all this was that anybody at all could accuse anyone else of being a witch, without having to produce a shred of evidence. It was up to the accused to prove their innocence, which of course, was practically impossible. Allied to this was the fact that large sums of money could be earnt by being a witch hunter or pricker — anywhere between 50p and £1 per conviction.

Legend has it that Matthew Hopkins, one of the most celebrated witch hunters of his day, was the subject of an experiment into the trial by water method, after he retired, and was condemned and executed as a wizard himself. He is credited with over 400 witch hangings, and 60 in one year alone in his own county, Essex.

Witchcraft was declared heresy by Pope Innocent VIII in a papal bull in 1484, and was made a capital offence in Britain in 1563. The Act was repealed in 1736. During this time about 200,000 'witches' were put to death by hanging, burning or torture in western Europe. Some of these were wise men and healers, similar to the legendary Merlin; but they all became witches according to the papal bull.

During this discussion of the mandrake plant, we have wandered slightly off course. To return once more to our central theme, let us consider afresh that the mandrake is a member of the potato family. Curiously enough, two other plants in the same family have also been credited with aphrodisiacal qualities — peppers and tomatoes.

5 Peppers, Tomatoes and Potatoes

I can find no exceptionally interesting stories connected with peppers, but they always seem to be included in aphrodisiacal lists, perhaps because of their exotic nature. The olden-day name for a tomato was a 'love apple'. Tomatoes were brought into Europe from Mexico at the end of the sixteenth century, and in Elizabethan times were looked upon mainly as an aphrodisiac; they have only become popular in Britain during the last fifty years or so, although they have been cultivated widely in Italy from about 1600 for use with spaghetti. Could this have been the start of the Italians' reputation as 'Latin Lovers'?

Mandrakes, peppers and tomatoes are all members of the potato family. Is this a coincidence? What of the humble potato itself? Potatoes are considered to be native to the Peruvian-Bolivian Andes, and are now one of the main food crops of the world. They were cultivated in South America as early as 150 AD, and probably comprised many varieties, as they still do in that area. They were introduced into Europe by certain Spanish adventurers during the second half of the sixteenth century, and in 1584 Sir Walter Raleigh took some tubers to Ireland.

They did not immediately find favour, and were initially used as aphrodisiacs. In fact, in the sixteenth century they were sold as such to unwitting recipients, reputedly for over £250 per pound. To understand the enormity of that price, consider that in those times a chicken would have cost one penny, a loaf of bread 1½p, a labourer earnt about £12 a year, and best beef was around 1½p a pound! You could say that potatoes were costing the equivalent of £6,000 an ounce nowadays.

In 1719 it was written that potatoes 'are of less note than

horseradish, radish scorzoners, beets and skirrets'. (Skirret had been cultivated for a long time in France and England, and was still being eaten in the twentieth century. Its value consists in its dahlia-like bundle of fleshy roots, which are 'greyish in colour and sweet flavoured when properly cooked'.)

In 1728 they were forbidden by law in Scotland, because the potato was an unholy plant of the nightshade family and not mentioned in the Bible. This was probably the culmination of over a hundred years of superstition towards the potato, when amongst other beliefs it was thought to thrive best if planted in the 'dark of moon', as long as it was not on Good Friday, when a poor crop would result.

By the end of the seventeenth century, potatoes were a major crop in Ireland. By the end of the eighteenth century they were a major crop in Europe generally, and in Germany and the West of England in particular. The Irish economy became dependent on it. Potatoes continued to spread both in western and eastern hemispheres, during the early part of the nineteenth century, until the failures of the Irish crops in 1845 and 1846, due to late blight, when more caution was shown towards the planting of it, especially because of the famine that followed.

During this time Europe's population increased at a rate hitherto unknown. This was not due to declines in death rates as there was no real advance in medical science at this time. Nevertheless, even with the heavy emigrations from Europe to the Americas the population exploded. And when did it explode most? Yes, you have guessed it. Between 1801 and 1901 the population increased in the UK from 11 million to 38 million, and in Germany from 25 million to 56 million! The two countries which ate the most potatoes had the largest population increases. Admittedly there was a slight decline in infant mortality at this time, but not enough to justify the increase.

Are potatoes really an aphrodisiac? Is there a connection between the fact that Sir Walter Raleigh took the potato to Ireland, that the staple diet of the Irish is said to be potatoes, and that the Irish have one of the largest birth rates? One may argue that lack of birth control is the major cause of this, but that is because we look at it from a modern viewpoint.

How would the Irish have seen it at the time? They were brought up knowing that potatoes were an aphrodisiac. They must have been if they commanded such a high price. We also know that potatoes were certainly not being eaten widely by 1719, over a hundred years later. During this time production was obviously rising, and the price becoming far far cheaper. It is also obvious that any Irish peasant who had easy access to potatoes and was convinced that if he ate one it would improve his virility would then go out to prove it! Although the aphrodisiacal qualities of the potato have long been forgotten by the Irish, it has certainly become inherent in their make-up, and must be considered as one of the reasons for the size of their families.

Potatoes were introduced into North America in the seventeenth century. Both there and in Europe it used to be carried in the pocket as a guard against rheumatism and sciatica, although in Holland it had to be stolen first. It was also believed that if warts were rubbed with a raw potato which is then hidden or buried, the wart will disappear as the potato rots.

Returning to Ireland again, it was also believed there to help cure aches, sprains and broken bones, if the water in which the potatoes were boiled was rubbed on the affected area. However, if you were to wash in this water, it would *cause* warts.

Poteen or Potheen is the name for an Irish whiskey produced from an illicit still, and made from potatoes. Too much of this is meant to make you blind — Poteen, that is!

6 Other Aphrodisiacs

BLOOD

Blood has always been believed to increase sexual power. Roman patricians who felt their sexual powers waning used to go into the arenas to drink the blood of the defeated gladiators. Daniel Beckler declared positively in London in an authoritive publication in 1660 that efficient love philtres can be made from human blood.

HONEY

'The nectar of the Gods' is extremely nutritious and for many years has also been believed to hold aphrodisiacal qualities. Amongst its followers have been Galen, Ovid and Sheikh Nefzawi, who was the author of *The Perfumed Garden*. Before sugar became widely available in Europe from the sixteenth century onwards, honey was virtually the sole sweetening agent.

LOBSTER

The lobster is considered to be an aphrodisiac purely because of the 'fish' association with Aphrodite. Anything that came from the sea is associated with Aphrodite and her love powers. Lobster was also described as an aphrodisiac by Henry Fielding in *Tom Jones* and by many other writers.

OYSTERS

Again there is the 'fish' connection. Oysters are one of the most famous of aphrodisiacs, are easily digested, and were used by many famous lovers including Casanova, who reputedly ate fifty of them every day for breakfast. There are numerous species and they are exceedingly prolific. British oysters were very highly prized by the Romans.

CAVIARE

Caviare is considered an aphrodisiac on three counts: 1) because of the amount of protein it contains; 2) because of its place in the reproductive cycle; 3) because of the 'fish' association. It is the roe of the sturgeon and other large fish of eastern European lakes and rivers, which have been pressed and salted.

EELS

Three reasons again, although slightly different. The first reason is the 'fish' power. The second is the excitant effect it has on the bladder, and the third is the phallic-like shape.

BLACK CHOW MEAT

This was eaten every day by General Chang Chung-Ch'ang, a

Chinese warlord who died in 1935, and was reputed to have taken on whole brothels at a time. He was also called '72 Cannon Chang' because his 'manhood' was supposed to have equalled 72 silver dollars in length and breadth, which may have been a slight exaggeration, and is certainly mind-boggling when one considers that if 72 dollars were stacked in a single column they would measure approximately 63×4 cm ($25 \times 1\frac{1}{2}$ inches)! He thought he owed his prowess to the Chow Meat.

PEACHES

In China the peach is regarded as an emblem of long life and immortality. The Arabs, as well as the Chinese, considered the deep downy-lined cleft of the peach as symbolic of the female genitalia, and its sweet juices as the efflux. Peach blossom is the emblem of a bride. A 'Peach House' used to be common slang for a brothel, in England, and the term 'peach' has been used for many years to describe a pretty or sexually appealing girl. In Japan it is also regarded as a symbol of fertility. In a more mundane mood, peach wood was occasionally used as a divining rod in the north of England, and was held in high esteem as such. The Navaho Indians used dried peaches as a purgative, and in Italy they believed that warts could be cured if peach leaves were buried. In Texas the leaves boiled in water were thought to be good for upset stomachs.

GARLIC

Garlic is found in most parts of the world, and is looked upon universally as an antiseptic and preventative of disease. It has long been regarded as a powerful aphrodisiac by both eastern and western cultures, and also by the Romans and Greeks. Roman soldiers ate garlic in the belief that it would give them courage in battle. It was introduced into Britain in the early sixteenth century.

TRUFFLES

These are an edible fungi found mainly in central and southern Europe, and usually found under oak trees. They are shaped like petals, with a black warty exterior, and a rich flavour. They are very high in protein. There are no positive indications on the ground surface as to where they are to be found, apart from a very slight odour. Pigs are best for sniffing them out, but dogs are also used. Amongst the devotees of its aphrodisiacal properties have been Rabelais, Casanova, Marquis de Sade, Napoleon and Madame Pompadour. They were much esteemed by the Romans, and have been used in cookery in France and Italy since the sixteenth century.

ASPARAGUS

Asparagus contains a diuretic which stimulates the kidneys, increases the amount of urine excreted, and excites the urinary passages. It was much valued by the Romans, and has been grown in Britain for at least 350 years. It has also got a sexy shape.

GINSENG

Called by the Chinese 'the elixir of life', it has been used as an aphrodisiac for over 5,000 years. Medical opinion is deeply divided over the merits of ginseng. Some Russian experimenters in recent years claim that it increases sexual energy and has a general healing and rejuvenating effect on the body. It is the root of a plant (the Panax) found in N. China, Korea, Nepal, Canada, and eastern USA. The Chinese and Korean variety (*Panax schinseng*) is considered to be better than the N. American (*Panax quinquefolium*). The name comes from the Chinese *jên shên*, which means 'image of man', which in turn comes from the shape of the root which resembles the figure of a man, and has sometimes been confused with the mandrake because of this. The root is powdered and taken in tea or wine. To obtain the full benefits, the whole of the root should be used.

AVOCADO PEARS

These have always had an air of mysticism about them, perhaps because of their exotic nature, perhaps because of the number of vitamins and minerals they contain. They are very high in vitamin E, and a good source of protein, vitamin C, the B vitamins and iron.

ALCOHOL

Treat with care! A glass or two is ideal for losing one's inhibitions, but an unconscious female or flaccid male may easily result from an excess. As the porter said in Shakespeare's *Macbeth*, alcohol 'provokes the desire, but it takes away the performance'.

PERFUMES

Artificial odours, in the form of perfumes, have been manufactured throughout the ages by many civilisations, including the ancient Chinese, the Egyptians, the Hindus, the Israelites, the Carthaginians, the Greeks and the Romans, to try to make themselves more appealing to the opposite sex.

Nowadays, not only will they make any man climb mountains and risk imminent death in order to give a sweet-smelling lovely a box of chocolates, but they will also make any woman available to the man who uses a certain type of aftershave. Or so the television informs us. As the television is never wrong, let us take a closer look at a few of the main ingredients of the most famous perfumes based on animal sources, and see exactly where they come from.

The most provocative smell used in perfumes is musk.

MUSK

Musk is of great value in the manufacture of a great variety of perfumes, and comes from the male Musk Deer. This is a small Himalayan animal, which stands about 50–60 cm (20–24 in) high at the shoulder, and carries a small pouch in its abdominal region into which it secretes a reddish-brown substance commonly known as musk. Musk is believed to have aphrodisiacal properties and also to be a stimulant, and is chemically related to the human sex hormones.

As with the rhinoceros, this animal was in danger of becoming extinct through wholesale slaughter for this substance, although nowadays the active ingredient, muscone, is manufactured synthetically.

AMBERGRIS

Ambergris is a grey or blackish fatty substance with ruddy marble like veins running through it. It is derived from the intestines of the sperm whale, and is found floating in tropical seas, or thrown up on the shore. One of the largest masses found was one off the Bahamas weighing about 226 kg (500 lb).

CIVET

Civet is a yellowish substance with the consistency of butter, which is accumulated in two large glands near the anus of the civet cat, or member of the same genus of small carnivorous animals. This secretion is used to mark territories, and the musky scented substance is collected several times weekly by the keeper of captive animals, for the perfume trade. Shakespeare was obviously well acquainted with its reputation when he wrote in *King Lear*: 'Give me an ounce of civet, good apothecary, to sweeten my imagination.'

CASTOR

This is a reddish-brown oily substance obtained from the dried glands of the skin covering the end of the penis of a beaver. These glands used also to be cut up and soaked in spirit to form a stimulant.

Having read the foregoing can we really say we have progressed much further than Pliny, Tung P'in, or the Arunta Australians?

We have now covered all the main aphrodisiacs used throughout the centuries, the majority of which are still looked upon as such. But what about this century? Are there any new aphrodisiacs? Almost every week we see a new kind of fruit or vegetable for sale in the shops, but no extravagant claims accompany them. It appears that for the moment we have exhausted the supply of non-scientific aphrodisiac foods. Is there anything the twentieth century has to offer us, aphrodisiacally speaking, from a scientific basis? Happily the answer is 'yes'. It is the discovery of vitamin E.

7 Vitamin E

This chapter of the story is not meant to be an authoritative or medical paper on vitamin E. It is a mixture of facts and theories. The truth is that very little is known in depth about this vitamin, and association with both rejuvenation and sexual enhancement theories has probably helped to hinder the amount of progress that could have been made in this field.

Another reason is that a deficiency of vitamin E does not appear to cause any specific disease, as is the case with other vitamins. We all know, for instance, that scurvy and beri beri are caused by deficiencies of vitamins C and B_1 respectively. This means that vitamin E has never had the impact of these other vitamins, and the interpretation of the results of various experiments over the years with vitamin E have caused continuing controversy amongst the medical profession.

One thing seems certain, though, and that is that the amount of vitamin E we obtain from food (and that is the only way we obtain it) has slowly been declining during this century due to modern methods of food processing. For instance, one of the best sources of vitamin E, as you will see later, is wheat germ. This is removed before the grain is ground in order to produce white bread. In fact, so many vitamins are discarded or destroyed during this process that a law was passed requiring vitamins B_1 and B_2, nicotinic acid, iron and calcium to be added. However, no provision was made for vitamin E, and the result is that white bread is now almost totally devoid of this vitamin. Large losses of vitamin E are also caused during modern food processing methods, particularly with respect to vegetables, from which the bulk of our vitamin E could be obtained.

It would appear then most likely that the majority of people in this country have insufficient vitamin E in their diet, but do not realise it, because they do not appear to suffer any visibly harmful effects. On the other hand, it must be said that some people say that in a well nourished adult there *should* be enough vitamin E to last several months, and there *should* be sufficient in a normal diet to satisfy the recommended dosage. However, as will be seen later, there is no definite recommended amount laid down by any country.

What you have to decide for yourself after reading the following information is whether you think there is any possibility at all that by stepping up your vitamin E intake your actual health and performance *might* improve, or not. If you think there is a chance, you will be shown how to increase the amounts of vitamin E you consume from everyday foods, without having to take recourse to tablets.

Vitamin E is not destroyed by cooking. It is fat-soluble, is absorbed throught the lymph, is stored in the liver, and is found in most of our organs such as the heart, spleen, liver, kidneys, lungs, pancreas, and muscles. The highest levels are in the adrenal glands, the pituitary and the testes.

It is found in every cell in our bodies, and is believed by some to slow down the ageing process, because it acts as an anti-oxidant. What happens is that the tissues in our bodies, particularly the unsaturated fats, are slowly destroyed by oxidisation. (An unsaturated fat is one where there is room in the molecule for another element such as oxygen or hydrogen. If it takes on oxygen it becomes oxidised, and if it takes on hydrogen it is hydrogenated — in other words, saturated.) Vitamin E helps to protect unsaturated fats from oxidisation, and thus from the ageing process. It does not prevent it, it only slows the rate of oxidisation down. Incidentally, when we talk of 'fats' we do not mean fat people. *All* humans have fat.

This ageing process happens to every part of our bodies.

Obviously, as far as the human life cycle is concerned, it will take a lifetime for these tissues to be sufficiently worn out so as not to sustain life any longer, unless death is caused by the premature failure of an essential organ, or through some outside interference. The rate of this ageing process varies from person to person — some people die in their seventies, some in their eighties, some in their nineties, and a few live to a hundred or more. It also varies from organ to organ. For instance, our first teeth only last a few years before being replaced with 'permanent' ones, which again start to decay and fall out from around the age of forty. It is a well-known fact that eyesight starts to deteriorate from the age of forty, our hearing generally becomes worse as we get older, and the hairline can start to recede from any age. As far as sex is concerned, how many of us are as active now as we were twenty or thirty years ago?

The questions we now have to ask ourselves are as follows.

1) Is it possible that, as Vitamin E is an anti-oxidant, if the level of vitamin E in the body is increased it will slow down the ageing process slightly, or, in the case of the sexual organs, help to rejuvenate them?

2) Is it a coincidence that the areas of the body where vitamin E is found in the greatest quantities all have sexual associations?

The presence of vitamin E was discovered at the University of California in 1922, when a group of research scientists fed a colony of rats on a special diet containing all the essential nutrients known to man. The rats behaved in a normal manner in every respect, apart from the females whose foetuses died before birth, and were reabsorbed, and the males who eventually became sterile. Fresh lettuce, dried alfalfa, meat, oats, wheat and milk were added to the same diet, and the rats then started to reproduce normally. Obviously something in the added foods redressed the balance, and the researchers assumed it was an as yet undiscovered essential nutrient, and thought it was probably a vitamin. They eventually identified this missing ingredient as a fat-soluble alcohol, and named it Tocopherol. This was formed from the Greek word *Tocos* meaning childbirth, and *Phero* meaning to bring forth or deliver. It was also given the letter 'E' as a classification, because this was the next available letter for vitamins.

By 1938 Tocopherol, or vitamin E, had been synthesised in the laboratory and a multitude of experiments began on rabbits, rats, chickens, dogs, sheep and cattle to see what happened when differing amounts of vitamin E were administered, and also none at all.

The results of these experiments varied tremendously, and led to any number of conclusions. For instance, with male rats, when vitamin E was withheld, their livers degenerated as did the sperm-producing cells of their testicles. Some chickens developed brain damage, muscular non-coordination and paralysis, and calves developed heart disease. It was thought that a deficiency in humans might be the cause of impotence and sterility in men, continual abortions in women, muscular weakness in both sexes, and also a major factor in coronary heart disease. The saying that 'fish give you brains' probably also came from the brain damage to chickens, as fish contains approximately ten times as much vitamin E as red meat.

Many experiments have been carried out over the years to see if extra vitamin E given to humans improved any of the conditions, but no conclusive evidence has been forthcoming. One reason put forward for this was that in normal circumstances the average human diet should contain sufficient vitamin E for our needs. However, the recommended dosage varies tremendously, and is based primarily upon the amount of fat we eat.

Dr Horwitt, head of the Biochemical Research Laboratories at the Elgin State Hospital in Illinois, was commissioned by the US National Research Council in 1967, to find out what happened to people if they were given a diet which contained only one third of the vitamin E found in a typical American diet. The result showed that the men and women subjects appeared to be as normal in every respect as those which had been fed on ordinary diets, even though their blood plasma alpha-tocopherol red blood cells only lived for an average of 110 days instead of 120. Dr Horwitt's conclusion was that humans only need a relatively small amount of vitamin E, and this should be adequately provided in our normal diet. He conceded that in exceptional circumstances a deficiency of vitamin E may possibly cause disease, but it was most unlikely to occur.

On the other hand, there are many doctors who profoundly disagree with this.

Commencing with the discovery in 1946, by the Shute brothers, Dr Evan and Dr Wilfred Shute, that vitamin E is able to dissolve fresh preformed blood clots, they have continued their research at the Shute Foundation for Medical Research in Canada, and claim that a larger dose of vitamin E also helps to combat many other complaints, including: skin problems, varicose veins, arthritis, diabetes, heart disease and several sexual problems. Many other doctors have carried out similar research, and agree with them. Dr A. Ochsner with regard to thrombosis, Dr Lambert with fatigue, Dr Livingstone and Dr Jones, in 1958, and Dr Haeger, in 1974, for Intermittent Claudication (a painful condition of the leg arteries), Dr Butturini for diabetes, Dr Burgess and Dr Pritchard for nerve root pain, and so on . . .

On the sexual side, Dr J. Milton reported that almost half of his fifty patients who were treated with a relatively small extra amount of vitamin E twice daily developed a higher density of spermatozoa in their semen, and most of the rest benefited with an increased volume of seminal fluid. Dr Lindner claimed that in many cases he was able to increase the sperm count in men

37

who had previously been unable to produce normal spermatozoa, by administering a slightly larger dose of vitamin E. Dr Evan Shute stated that he found a lack of vitamin E led to a wasting away of the reproductive parts in men, eventually leading to complete sterility. He further claimed that if extra vitamin E were taken both virility and fertility returned.

There appears to be no evidence that vitamin E helps to combat sterility in women, but quite a substantial amount regarding the prevention of miscarriages. Dr Bayer, for example, conducted experiments on many couples able to conceive, but where miscarriages always resulted. He found that if both the men and the women took extra specified amounts of Vitamin E for three months before conception, the abortion rate dropped to just 2½ per cent. Amongst another group of people who normally only managed to give birth in roughly one in three conceptions, there was a 100 per cent record, with 41 pregnancies, and 41 babies successfully delivered.

Both the Shute Foundation and Dr H. Gozan of New York, amongst others, claim success in treating the troublesome symptoms associated with the menopause, and also with easing menstruation problems.

Nevertheless there is also a mountain of opinion that says there is absolutely no truth in these assertions. In 1973 the National Research Council of the USA stated that following a full investigation of all the available data and results of various tests that had been carried out, there was no evidence to suggest that any of these claims were true. It stated that 'many of the claims made for vitamin E are based on misinterpretations of research on experimental animals', and that the claim that it enhances sexual potency stems from the experiments that show it was only *among* the factors required to prevent sterility in male rats and to permit normal pregnancy in female rats. It goes on to say that the widespread distribution of vitamin E in vegetable oils, cereal grains, and animal fats makes it extremely unlikely that any humans ever suffer from a deficiency of vitamin E. But are statements like these part of a deliberate plot to play down the effects of vitamin E, and thus avert a population explosion in the Western World which would equal that of the East? I leave you to decide.

One last thought. Have you noticed that the levels of vitamin E are never mentioned among the list of added vitamins and minerals on the sides of breakfast cereal packets? Could this be because there might be a potential loss in sales if mothers thought that by allowing their children to have extra bowls of breakfast cereals they might be turning them into sex maniacs?

If, after reading the background to vitamin E, you think there may be some truth in the claims of its adherents, then I suggest you concentrate on eating vitamin E rich food. The daily requirements of vitamin E are put anywhere between 3 and 30 mg. The following tables list the amounts of vitamin E (per 25 g/1 oz) in foods which contain the highest levels of this vitamin. As alpha-tocopherol occurs with most frequency in vegetable oils and cereals, which are also high in calories, I have also listed the amounts of calories present, the number of ounces of the food that would have to be eaten to provide 5 mg of vitamin E, and the total number of calories that would be involved. The table is not shown as a guide for your eating habits, but merely to emphasise the differing amounts of vitamin E in various foods, and to bring this home to you by showing how much of a certain food it would be necessary to eat to achieve 5 mg. I have chosen this figure as this is just above the minimum suggested requirement given above. I would not, even in my wildest dreams, suggest, or care to imagine, anyone eating 2.4 kg (85 oz) or 42 sausages, which would total 6,078 calories. It is just there for comparison purposes with other foods such as caviare — 65 g (2½ oz) and 151 calories!

The average daily diet probably contains somewhere between 5 and 20 mg of vitamin E per day. Large doses are not meant to be harmful; in fact up to 1,000 mg per day is considered to be perfectly safe, and 3–4,000 mg are frequently given under medical supervision.

POLYUNSATURATED FATS

With increasing concern over the amounts of cholesterol consumed and the link with heart disease, polyunsaturated fats are becoming more and more popular. Their use alters radically the amount of vitamin E needed by each individual. The more polyunsaturated fats you eat, the more vitamin E will be needed. This is usually compensated for by the fact that polyunsaturated fats are very high in vitamin E content anyway.

However, there is a difference between the amounts of vitamin E in different vegetable oils, as illustrated below.

Oil	Vit. E per 25 g/oz
Wheat germ oil	37.8 mg
Sunflower seed	13.9 mg
Cotton seed	11.1 mg
Safflower seed	11.0 mg
Palm	7.3 mg
Rapeseed	5.3 mg
Peanut	3.7 mg
Maize	3.2 mg
Soyabean	2.9 mg
Saturated fats { Olive	1.5 mg
Coconut	0.2 mg

VITAMIN E TABLE

Food	mg of vit. E per 25 g/oz	calories per 25 g/oz	g/oz to provide 5 mg vit. E	calories in 5 mg of vit. E
Wheat germ oil	37.78	256	6/ 0.2	52
Sunflower seed	13.83	256	11/ 0.4	102
Polyunsaturated margarine	7.10	104	20/ 0.7	73
Cobnuts (hazelnuts)	5.97	108	26/ 0.9	98
Cod liver oil	5.68	256	26/ 0.9	231
Almonds	5.68	161	26/ 0.9	145
Marzipan	2.59	126	57/ 2.0	252
Peanuts	2.30	162	62/ 2.2	357
Cod roe (fried)	1.96	58	74/ 2.6	151
Brazil nuts	1.85	176	77/ 2.7	476
Canned tuna in oil	1.79	83	79/ 2.8	233
Potato crisps	1.73	152	82/ 2.9	441
Olive oil	1.45	256	99/ 3.5	896
Mayonnaise	1.39	200	102/ 3.6	720
Peanut butter	1.34	177	108/ 3.8	673
French dressing	1.11	187	128/ 4.5	842
Blackberries	0.99	9	145/ 5.1	46
Avocado pears	0.91	64	156/ 5.5	352
Muesli	0.91	107	156/ 5.5	589
Sponge cake (with oil)	0.77	86	184/ 6.5	559
Asparagus	0.71	6	201/ 7.1	43
Iced fruit cake	0.68	100	210/ 7.4	740
Choux pastry	0.60	94	238/ 8.4	790
All Bran	0.57	71	249/ 8.8	625
Butter (salted)	0.57	210	249/ 8.8	1848
Spinach	0.57	9	249/ 8.8	80
Weetabix	0.51	99	278/ 9.8	971
Flaky pastry	0.51	161	278/ 9.8	1578
Parsley, raw	0.51	6	278/ 9.8	59
Grapenuts	0.45	100	318/11.2	1120
Rock cakes	0.45	112	318/11.2	1255
Sponge pudding	0.45	98	318/11.2	1098
Eggs	0.45	42	332/11.7	492
Salmon, canned	0.43	44	332/11.7	515
Lobster	0.43	34	332/11.7	398
Rich fruit cake	0.40	94	354/12.5	1175
Short crust pastry (plain pie crust) (cooked)	0.40	150	354/12.5	1875
Tomato sauce	0.40	25	354/12.5	313
Cornish pastie (meat patty)	0.37	95	386/13.6	1292

Food	mg of vit. E per 25 g/oz	calories per 25 g/oz	g/oz to provide 5 mg vit. E	calories in 5 mg of vit. E
Sausage roll	0.37	136	386/13.6	1850
Bolognese sauce	0.37	40	389/13.6	544
Mussels	0.34	25	417/14.7	368
Ready Brek	0.34	113	417/14.7	1662
Gingerbread	0.34	106	417/14.7	1559
Eclairs	0.34	107	417/14.7	1573
Lamb sweetbreads, fried	0.34	65	417/14.7	956
Tomatoes	0.34	4	417/14.7	59
Xmas (rich fruit) pudding	0.31	86	459/16.2	1394
Brains, boiled	0.31	43	459/16.2	697
Broccoli tops (greens)	0.31	6	459/16.2	98
Spring greens (cabbage)	0.31	3	459/16.2	49
Shredded Wheat	0.28	101	507/17.9	1808
Lemon meringue pie	0.28	92	507/17.9	1947
Skate, fried	0.28	57	507/17.9	1021
Kedgeree (smoked fish and rice)	0.28	43	507/17.9	770
Parsnips	0.28	16	507/17.9	287
Watercress	0.28	4	507/17.9	72
Blackcurrants	0.28	8	507/17.9	144
Double (heavy) cream	0.34	127	507/17.9	2274
Stilton cheese	0.28	132	507/17.9	2363
Cream cheese	0.28	125	507/17.9	2238
Halibut	0.28	38	507/17.9	681
Parmesan cheese	0.25	116	567/20.0	2320
Quiche Lorraine	0.25	111	567/20.0	2220
Brussels sprouts	0.25	6	567/20.0	120
Curried meat	0.24	46	593/20.9	962
Oysters	0.24	15	593/20.9	314
Fish paste	0.24	49	593/20.9	1025
Mince pies (mincemeat tarts)	0.23	124	618/21.8	2704
Apple crumble (crisp)	0.23	59	618/21.8	1287
Custard tart (pie)	0.23	82	618/21.8	1788
Cheddar cheese	0.23	120	618/21.8	2616
Edam cheese	0.23	87	618/21.8	1897
Scotch egg	0.23	80	618/21.8	1744
Sardines	0.23	61	618/21.8	1330
Whelks	0.23	26	618/21.8	567
Leeks	0.23	7	618/21.8	153
Peppers	0.23	5	618/21.8	109
Walnuts	0.23	150	618/21.8	3270
Tomato chutney (pickle)	0.23	44	618/21.8	960

Food	mg of vit. E per 25 g/oz	calories per 25 g/oz	g/oz to provide 5 mg vit. E	calories in 5 mg of vit. E
(Ground) corned beef	0.22	62	646/22.8	1414
Blue cheese	0.20	101	708/25.0	2303
Pizza	0.20	67	708/25.0	1528
Sardines, canned	0.20	36	708/25.0	821
Mustard and cress (mustard greens)	0.20	3	708/25.0	69
Damsons	0.20	11	708/25.0	251
Plums	0.20	11	708/25.0	251
Sultanas (golden raisins)	0.20	71	708/25.0	1619
Coconut	0.20	100	708/25.0	2280
Rice Krispies	0.17	100	836/29.5	2950
Jam tarts	0.17	109	836/29.5	3216
Treacle tarts (molasses crumb tarts)	0.17	106	836/29.5	3127
Baked beans	0.17	19	836/29.5	561
Cheese sauce	0.17	56	836/29.5	1652
White sauce	0.17	43	836/29.5	1269
Beefburgers, fried	0.16	75	887/31.3	2348
Cod	0.16	27	887/31.3	846
Special K	0.14	102	1015/35.8	3652
Crispbread	0.14	110	1015/35.8	3938
Evaporated milk	0.14	45	1015/35.8	1611
Single (light) cream	0.14	61	1015/35.8	2184
Carrots	0.14	6	1015/35.8	215
Lettuce	0.14	4	1015/35.8	144
Sweetcorn (corn)	0.14	35	1015/35.8	1253
Chestnuts	0.14	49	1015/35.8	1755
Chocolate	0.14	150	1015/35.8	5370
Beef, fatty	0.14	120	1015/35.8	4296
Cauliflower cheese	0.11	33	1290/45.5	1502
Welsh rarebit (cheese toast)	0.11	104	1290/45.5	4732
Cornflakes	0.11	100	1290/45.5	4550
Heart	0.11	68	1290/45.5	3094
Kidney	0.11	44	1290/45.5	2002
Oxtail	0.11	69	1290/45.5	3140
Ice cream	0.11	48	1290/45.5	2184
Cocoa powder	0.11	89	1290/45.5	4050
Egg custard	0.09	34	1576/55.6	1891
Pancakes (crepes)	0.09	89	1576/55.6	4949
Trifle (tipsy cake)	0.09	46	1576/55.6	2558
Yorkshire (batter) pudding	0.09	62	1576/55.6	3448

Food	mg of vit. E per 25 g/oz	calories per 25 g/oz	g/oz to provide 5 mg vit. E	calories in 5 mg of vit. E
Macaroni cheese	0.09	50	1576/55.6	2780
Brisket	0.09	93	1576/55.6	5171
Mince (ground meat) and most (solid) red meat	0.09	80	1576/55.6	4448
Liver	0.09	66	1576/55.6	3670
Tongue	0.09	84	1576/55.6	4671
Moussaka	0.09	56	1576/55.6	3114
Herring	0.09	67	1576/55.6	3726
Kippers (kippered herrings)	0.09	59	1576/55.6	3281
Gooseberries	0.09	11	1576/55.6	612
Grapefruit	0.09	7	1576/55.6	390
Loganberries (black raspberries)	0.09	5	1576/55.6	278
Raspberries	0.09	8	1576/55.6	445
Salami	0.08	140	1772/62.5	8750
Shepherds (cottage) pie	0.08	34	1772/62.5	2125
Sausages	0.07	85	2027/71.5	6078
French (snap) beans	0.06	2	2364/83.4	167
Apples	0.06	10	2364/83.4	834
Bananas	0.06	14	2364/83.4	1168
Oranges	0.06	8	2364/83.4	668
Rhubarb	0.06	2	2364/83.4	167
Strawberries	0.06	8	2364/83.4	668
Tomato juice, canned	0.06	5	2364/83.4	417
Bread sauce	0.06	32	2364/83.4	2669
Milk	0.56 per pint (0.22 per cup)			

Almost all other foods contain less vitamin E per 25 g/oz, and a
fair percentage of those none at all.

The following table has been compiled from the top foods in the previous pages, in which 5 mg of vitamin E may be obtained in a day by eating reasonable quantities, whilst keeping the total number of calories under control.

Food	g/oz	Calories
Asparagus	201/ 7.1	43
Blackberries	145/ 5.1	46
Spring greens (cabbage)	459/16.2	49
Wheat germ oil	6/ 0.2	52
Tomatoes	417/14.7	59
Spinach	249/ 8.8	80
Broccoli tops (greens)	459/16.2	98
Cobnuts (hazelnuts)	26/ 0.9	98
Peppers	618/21.8	109
Brussels sprouts	567/20.0	120
Blackcurrants (black currants)	507/17.9	144
Almonds	26/ 0.9	145
Cod roe and caviare	74/ 2.6	151
Leeks	618/21.8	153
Canned tuna	79/ 2.8	233
Marzipan	57/ 2.0	252
Parsnips	507/17.9	287
Oysters	592/20.9	314
Avocado pears	160/ 5.5	352
Peanuts	62/ 2.2	357
Mussels	417/14.7	368
Lobster	332/11.7	398

The above table may be split further into food groupings, in order, as follows.

Fish	Fruit	Vegetables	Nuts
Cod roe/caviare	Blackberries	Asparagus	Cobnuts (hazelnuts)
Canned tuna	Tomatoes	Spring greens (cabbage)	Almonds
Oysters	Blackcurrants	Spinach	Peanuts
Mussels	Avocado pears	Broccoli tops (greens)	
Lobster		Peppers	
		Brussels sprouts	
		Leeks	
		Parsnips	

What do you notice? Our old friends are back again! The 'fish' association, including oysters, lobster and caviare — our direct line with Aphrodite. These also provide a very good source of protein. The fruit section contains tomatoes and avocado pears, and also provides a good source of vitamin C. Top of the vegetable section is asparagus, with peppers not far behind.

If we discount the nuts, which are very high in polyunsaturates, and will therefore need more vitamin E to protect against the oxidisation process, we are left with the fact that 53 per cent of the above foods were classified as aphrodisiacs. Looking back again to the previous table of order of merit, we see that the top two items are seasonal, the third would become very tiresome in those quantities throughout the year, and the fourth is almost all polyunsaturated fat. The top all-the-year-round food, then, is the tomato.

We have now come full circle. We have examined the aphrodisiacs of the past, looked at results of experiments carried out in this century, and married the two together.

Is it just a coincidence that a number of foods which have been thought of as aphrodisiacs for hundreds, sometimes thousands, of years, also contain the highest levels of vitamin E without being fattening? Is it a further coincidence that the top-all-the-year-round food, the tomato, is a member of the potato family, as are the legendary mandrake, and the pepper? Is the potato really an aphrodisiac also? What about Casanova with his fifty oysters for breakfast? Were they the secret of his success after all? I leave you to think about it, and continue in Part II with some recipes designed around the foods in question, some old and some new. For ease of reference, I have included both the total number of calories involved in the meals, and the amount of mg of vitamin E, where possible.

Meanwhile, here are some well-known proverbs for you to ponder on.

A Bad Workman Blames His Tools.
A Bird In The Hand Is Worth Two In The Bush.
A Good Wife Makes A Good Husband.
A Man Can Do No More Than He Can.
A Man Is As Old As He Feels; A Woman Is As Old As She Looks.
A Short Life And A Gay One.
All Things Come To Those Who Wait.
Desires Are Nourished By Delays.
If At First You Don't Succeed, Try, Try, Try Again.
Kindle Not A Fire That You Cannot Extinguish.
When The Wine Is In, The Wit Is Out.

PART II –
THE RECIPES

Introduction

The figures shown for calories and vitamin E content after most of the following recipes are based upon average food weights, and because of this should only be taken as a general indication. The proportions given are for two servings.

SETTING THE SCENE

Eating in the correct surroundings is almost as important as the food you serve, and in some instances more important, because it is very difficult to be turned on physically if there is no mental stimulation. As an example, imagine you have been out for the day, and you decide to have a meal before returning home.

The only place that is open is Jack's Cafe. It does not look too dirty, although it is very difficult to see inside through the steamed-up windows. You and your partner go inside and find two spaces on the end green formica-topped table, which is already occupied by two men in donkey jackets. The menu is chalked on a blackboard on the wall, and the room appears to be filled with road sweepers, tramps and the entire work-force of the Gas Board, judging by the number of vans parked outside. The room is noisy and smoky, the table is fairly clean after the salt particles have been brushed aside, the cutlery is lightweight aluminium, the china is heavyweight clay. The meal you ordered, 'Sausage and Mash', which was the speciality of the day, was perfectly edible, and the coffee that followed was passable also. The only feelings you eventually leave the premises with are full ones in your stomach.

Now imagine the same beginning, but this time the only place open is a little French restaurant.

The lighting is low, the floor is thickly carpeted, and soft music plays in the background. The tables are intimate, laid with clean tablecloths, good quality cutlery, adorned with small bunches of flowers, and candles in decorative holders, which the attentive waiter lights immediately you are seated. You are each presented with a large menu, and choose 'Saucisses de Boeuf, et Pommes de Terre Purée' (sausage and mash). The food is exactly the same as that served in Jack's Cafe, but this time is presented on an attractively decorated oval plate, etc., etc . . . Hopefully you will leave the restaurant with more on your mind than a full stomach. Might one say baser thoughts?

The point of this story is to stress that it is no use cooking a sexy meal, and then dishing it up on the kitchen table, amongst a lot of clutter. You will be surprised how easily you can turn your dining room, or even your kitchen, if you normally eat there, into a cosy little French restaurant.

The first essential is background music. This can be provided either by a record player or by a cassette recorder, and the playing time should be sufficient that you do not have to jump up in the middle of your meal to turn the record or tape over.

The second essential is candlelight. With all the electric lighting off, and the table only illuminated by one or two candles, you will be able to imagine yourself anywhere. It may sound corny, but it works!

The next thing to concern yourself with is the choice of menu, and style of serving. It is best if this can be arranged so that you are away from the table for the minimum amount of time. This is done by having a mixture of cold courses prepared in advance, and hot dishes set on the table in tureens or on platters. Take the telephone off the hook, disconnect the doorbell, put the children to bed, chuck the cats out and get on with it.

One last thought. All pleasures become more appealing after a period of abstinence, and unfortunately as we become older this period lengthens. What might have been a thrice-nightly occurrence at twenty may have diminished to thrice-monthly by the age of fifty. This is called 'quality' and not 'quantity', and should be borne in mind when planning forward for a 'special' evening.

Make sure the dice are loaded in your favour as much as possible by ensuring that the body is capable of obeying the commands of the brain. Remember, there can be no Act without a Scene, so set yours properly, and the only things you will need to keep crossed will be your fingers!

GUIDE TO FOODS IN SEASON

Food	Spring	Summer	Autumn	Winter
Asparagus	███████			
Blackberries		██████	███	
Blackcurrants (currants)		███		
Broccoli	███████████████████████████			
Brussels sprouts		████████████████████		
Caviare	████████████████████████████			
Leeks	█████		███████████	
Lobster	███	██████████████████		
Mussels	█		████████████████████	
Oysters	██		██████████████████	
Parsnips	███		██████████████████	
Peppers	████████████████████████████			
Peaches	█████████████████████			
Spring greens (cabbage)	███			████████
Spinach		████		
Tomatoes	████████████████████████████			
Truffles	████████████████████████████			

Asparagus

Asparagus is in season from spring to summer and should be had as fresh as possible. Calculate on using 225 g of asparagus per person. The stalks should be green, and the tips firm and compact.

Undo the bundles and cut off any tough bottom ends and large scales that cling to the bottoms of the spears. Next, wash them carefully under cold running water, and cut into uniform lengths. Tie them into faggots, or small bundles. They should have two ties — one near the top, the other near the bottom.

Place upright in a saucepan of boiling salted water, with the heads just out of the water, because they require less cooking. Test the bottom ends of the stalks with the sharp point of a knife after about 30 minutes. Drain well when cooked.

Alternatively, the stalks may be peeled, in which case they should be lain horizontally in the saucepan, and will only take 15–20 minutes cooking time.

Asparagus may be used as an hors d'oeuvre appetizer, or as a vegetable accompanying meat or fish dishes.

ASPARAGUS WITH BUTTER
(*Asperges au Beurre*)

asparagus
pinch salt

pinch sugar
melted butter

Cook asparagus, or use canned or frozen. Drain well, season with salt and sugar, add melted butter.

ASPARAGUS SALAD

lettuce
asparagus
stuffed olives
hard-boiled (hard-cooked)
  eggs

tomato slices
green peppers, sliced
mayonnaise thinned with
  vinegar

Arrange the asparagus, olives, egg slices and tomato slices on the lettuce. Top with the slices of green peppers and garnish with the mayonnaise.

439 calories, 8.2 mg vitamin E, per person.

ASPARAGUS FINGERS

slices of toast cut into fingers
asparagus
butter

grated cheese
paprika
chopped parsley
pinch salt

Melt the butter with the salt, and heat the asparagus in it (either fresh cooked, frozen or canned). Cut into suitable lengths, and place upon fingers of toast. Sprinkle grated cheese over the top, and put under a medium grill and oven-broil to melt the cheese. Sprinkle with paprika pepper and chopped parsley. Serve at once on hot dishes.

ASPARAGUS POLONI
(*Asperges à la Polonaise*)

450 g (1 lb) asparagus
15 ml (1 tbls) fresh
   breadcrumbs
2 hard-boiled (hard-cooked)
   egg yolks, chopped
   (minced)

50 g (2 oz/¼ cup) butter
15 ml (1 tbls) chopped
   (minced) parsley

Cook the asparagus, drain, and put into a hot dish. Fry the breadcrumbs in butter, and sprinkle over the asparagus. Top with chopped (minced) egg yolks and parsley.

380 calories, 7.7 mg vitamin E, per person.

GRILLED (BROILED) ASPARAGUS WITH CHEESE (*Asperges Au Gratin*)

450 g (1 lb) asparagus
25 g (1 oz/¼ cup) flour
25 g (1 oz/2 tbls) butter

275 ml (½ pt/1¼ cups)
   milk
50 g (2 oz/½ cup) grated
   cheese

Cook the asparagus and place in a row on a fire-proof dish. Melt the butter, stir in the flour, cook a few minutes, then stir in the milk. Bring to the boil stirring constantly, and add half the cheese. Beat the sauce to get it smooth and shiny, then coat the asparatus — particularly the heads — and sprinkle the rest of the cheese over it. Place under a hot grill (broil) to brown. If any of the asparagus is not covered with the sauce, lay some foil over it for protection.

405 calories, 6.4 mg vitamin E, per person.

ASPARAGUS SOUP (*Crème d'Asperges*)

450 g (1 lb) asparagus or
   250 g (10 oz) can of
   asparagus
20 g (¾ oz/4 tsp) butter
20 g (¾ oz/1½ tbls flour)

425 ml (¾ pt/2 cups)
   chicken stock (broth)
½ onion
50 ml (2 fl oz/¼ cup) single
   (light) cream

Cut off the heads of the asparagus and cook them in a little of the stock until tender. Keep these for a garnish. Melt the butter in a saucepan, stir in the flour, gradually add the stock and bring to the boil. Put in the onion and asparagus cut into pieces, and simmer for approximately 30 minutes, or until tender. Pass through a sieve or put in a blender, reheat and season. Take off the heat, add the cream and asparagus heads, stir and serve.

ASPARAGUS WITH MOUSSELINE SAUCE (*Asperges Mousseline*)

450 g (1 lb) asparagus
60 ml (4 tbls) cream
15 g (½ oz/1 tbls) butter
2 egg yolks
10 ml (2 tsp) lemon juice

10 ml (2 tsp) stock or water
1 egg white, whisked
   (beaten)
salt
pepper

Cook asparagus normally, and arrange on hot dishes. Whilst the asparagus is cooking, place the cream, egg yolks, stock, salt and pepper into a bowl set into a saucepan of boiling water, and whisk (beat) until it thickens. Remove from the heat, whisk (beat) in the lemon juice and butter, and lastly fold in the egg white. Serve immediately with the asparagus.

Avocado Pears

Avocado pears are native to Mexico and surrounding areas, but are now grown in many other countries. They have a large stone in their centre, and the fruits vary a great deal in size. Test for ripeness by pressing the fleshy end very gently — it should yield slightly. They are usually eaten raw with salt, pepper and lemon juice, or with a salad dressing. Once they have been cut they tend to discolour very quickly. To overcome this, brush the cut faces with lemon juice.

AVOCADO PEARS WITH PRAWNS (SHRIMP)

1 large avocado pear
20 ml (4 tsp) prawns
10 ml (2 tsp) mayonnaise
lemon wedges
10 ml (2 tsp) tomato
ketchup (catsup)
cayenne pepper
lettuce

Cut the avocados in half with a sharp knife. Remove the stone, and brush the cut face of the avocado with lemon juice to stop it discolouring. Mix together with mayonnaise and tomato ketchup, then combine the prawns, ensuring that they are fully coated. Spoon into the pear halves, and sprinkle cayenne pepper over the top. Garnish with lettuce leaves and wedges of lemon. Serve with brown (whole wheat) bread and butter.

619 calories, 8.7 mg vitamin E, per person.

AVOCADO AND TUNA CREAM

1 ripe avocado
10 ml (2 tsp) lemon juice
50 g (2 oz) tuna
10 ml (2 tsp) mayonnaise

50 ml (2 fl oz/¼ cup)
  double (heavy) cream
salt
pepper

Cut the avocado in half, remove the stone and spoon out the flesh, keeping the skins intact. Mash the flesh with the lemon juice. Flake the tuna, combine with the mayonnaise, and add to the pear. Whip the fresh cream, and add this with the salt and pepper to the other ingredients. Pile back into the skins, and serve on a bed of lettuce, with brown (whole wheat) bread and butter, and lemon wedges as a garnish.

798 calories, 10.9 mg vitamin E, per person.

AVOCADO WITH
CARROT SALAD

225 g (½ lb) carrots
juice of 2 medium oranges
juice of ¼ lemon

salt and sugar to taste
1 avocado pear
4 anchovy fillets,
  drained

Wash, peel and grate the carrots. Cover with the orange and lemon juice, add sugar and salt to taste, and refrigerate overnight, or during the day, so that the carrots may absorb as much of the juice as possible. Quarter the avocado lengthwise, remove the stone, fill with the drained carrots, and top each with an anchovy fillet.

584 calories, 9.4 mg vitamin E, per person.

AVOCADO CITRUS SALAD

½ orange   lemon wedges
½ grapefruit   French dressing
1 avocado pear

Peel the orange, grapefruit and avocado, and cut into slices — half rounds. Arrange alternately around lemon wedges on a bed of lettuce, and sprinkle French dressing over the dish.

578 calories, 8.68 mg vitamin E, per person.

AVOCADO CREAM

1 avocado pear   2 anchovy fillets
30 ml (2 tbls) double (heavy)   lemon juce
  cream
salt, pepper

Cut the avocado in half, remove the stone, then spoon out the flesh into a bowl and mash. Try to leave the skins intact. Chop the anchovy fillets very finely and stir into the mashed avocados. Whip (beat) the cream, and combine with the other ingredients. Add a pinch of caster sugar, salt, pepper and lemon juice to taste. Pile back into the avocado skins, and sprinkle with paprika pepper.

652 calories, 8.78 mg vitamin E, per person.

Caviare

Caviare is the richest and the most delicate of hors d'oeuvres. Its price is always high. It should be served very simply, in a dish packed in ice, and accompanied by dark rye bread and lemon wedges. Alternatively, serve on shaped slices of toast, or on one of the commercially packaged canapé-type bases that may be purchased from the shops.

NATIVES (OYSTERS) WITH CAVIARE

This is a very luxurious hors d'oeuvres. On a tartlet-shaped base, place 15 ml (1 tbls) of caviare. Make a hollow in the centre, and place a fresh oyster in it. Season with a little pepper and a drop of lemon juice.

Lobster (Homard)

Chicken lobsters weigh 350–450 g (¾–1 lb), medium lobsters 450–700 g (1–1½ lb), and large or select ones 700–900 g (1½–2 lb) or heavier. They may be bought alive or already cooked. Do not overcook lobster in hot dishes.

BUYING ALIVE

The best weight is 450–700 g (1–1½ lb), which should give two servings. They should be active, and a mottled blue-green colour. There are two methods of cooking lobsters.

1) Bring 2.3 l (4 pt/10 cups) of water to the boil, and add 15 ml (1 tbls) salt. Pick up the lobster from behind the head, wash well, and plunge it head first into boiling water. Simmer until cooked.

2) Place in a large pan, cover with water, add the salt, bring slowly to the boil, then simmer until cooked. This is meant to be a more humane way of cooking the lobster, as it is sent to sleep and does not realise what is happening.

The length of time for cooking will depend on the size, but when cooked the shell should be coral pink or red. Rub the shells when cool with a little salad oil to brighten the colour.

BUYING COOKED

Cooked lobsters are sold whole or in halves, and should be red in colour. To test if the lobster was alive when cooked, straighten the tail and see if it springs back. It should also feel heavy for its size. 1.35 kg (3 lb) of cooked lobster in the shell should give about 175 g (6 oz) of meat. You can get the fishmonger to split the lobster and remove the intestinal cord so that you may then prepare it more easily. Cooked lobster may also be bought canned or frozen.

TO PREPARE

Remove the large claws by giving them a sharp twist, and then with a heavy weight crack open and remove the meat from the claws. Keep the small claws to use as a garnish. Cut off the head if you like. When it is cool, split the lobster from head to tail with a sharp knife, starting at the head end. Lift out the tail flesh from the lobster halves. Wash the shells and discard the narrow intestinal cord. Replace the sliced flesh in the cleaned shells. The meat in the claws is especially flavoursome. There is no dark meat on a lobster, but the bright red 'coral' found in female lobsters is most delicious. Serve with a green salad tossed in french dressing, and thinly sliced brown bread and butter.

LOBSTER SALAD (*Salade de Homard*)

Garnish the bottom of a serving bowl with roughly sliced lettuce, and cover with flaked lobster. Garnish directly upon the lobster with anchovy fillets, capers, stoned olives, slices or quarters of hard-boiled (hard-cooked) eggs etc., and make a border of radishes, small slices of cucumber etc. Serve with French dressing.

LOBSTER THERMIDOR
(*Homard Thermidor*)

1 lobster, cooked
1 small shallot
75 ml (3 fl oz/6 tbls) white
  wine
25 g (1 oz/2 tbls) butter
75 g (3 oz/¾ cup) grated
  cheese

White sauce
25 g (1 oz/¼ cup) flour
20 g (¾ oz/4 tsp) butter
125 ml (4 fl oz/½ cup) milk
2.5 ml (½ tsp) mixed
  mustard

Slit the lobster in half lengthwise, and remove the stomach and intestinal cord. Remove the meat from the shells, and cut into pieces. Chop (mince) the shallot finely, and place in a saucepan with the wine. Cook until the shallot is tender, and the wine has been reduced by half. Melt the butter and heat the meat very carefully in it. Make up a white sauce by melting the butter, adding flour, and then milk, in the usual fashion. Add to the sauce the mustard, half the cheese, the shallot and wine mixture, and stir. Then pour this over the lobster in butter, and mix carefully. Return to the shells, sprinkle with the remainder of the grated cheese, and brown under a pre-heated hot grill (in the broiler).

575 calories, 2.3 mg vitamin E, per person.

LOBSTER AMERICAINE
(*Homard à l'Americaine*)

1 medium to large cooked
  lobster
30 ml (2 tbls) olive oil
15 g (½ oz/1 tbls) butter

125 ml (4 fl oz/½ cup)
  white wine
15 ml (1 tbls) brandy
pinch of cayenne pepper
25 g (1 oz) tomato purée
  (paste)

Dice the onion finely, and skin and chop the tomatoes. Heat the olive oil and butter in a large frying pan, and then fry the onions, but do not brown. Add the skinned chopped tomatoes, tomato purée (paste), wine, brandy and cayenne pepper, and simmer for 10 minutes. Remove all the cooked lobster meat from the shell and claws. Slice or dice the meat, season and then add to the tomato mixture. Heat for 5 minutes.

SERVING

Either pour into two dishes, and serve with crisp toast, or, if served as a main course, spoon the mixture back into the lobster shell. Place on a dish and garnish with the small claws, watercress, wedges of lemon, or salad.

460 calories, 5.1 mg vitamin E, per person.

LOBSTER BISQUE (*Bisque de Homard*)

1 small cooked lobster
275 ml (½ pt/1¼ cups)
  water
5 ml (1 tsp) lemon juice
seasoning
25 g (1 oz/¼ cup) flour
275 ml (½ pt/1¼ cups)
  milk

25 g (1 oz/2 tbls) butter
30 ml (2 tbls) cream
25 g (1 oz) onion
25 g (1 oz) carrot
1 spring parsley
cayenne pepper

Remove the meat from the lobster, and cut into small pieces, saving a few tiny whole pieces for garnishing purposes.

Make 200 g (8 oz) bouillon by the following method.

Wash and crush the shell, and place in a saucepan with the water, lemon juice and seasoning. Bring to the boil and simmer gently for 30 minutes. Strain the liquid very carefully, and then add sufficient water to make back to 225 ml (8 fl oz/1 cup).

Heat the butter in a saucepan, stir in the flour and cook for a few minutes on a low heat. Slowly add the milk and the bouillon, stirring all the time, and simmer slowly until the mixture thickens. Add the lobster, onion, carrot and parsley, and simmer for a further 10 minutes. Remove from the heat and either: 1) strain through a sieve, pressing as much of the meat as possible through the sieve; or 2) blend in an electric blender until smooth. Season to taste. Add the cream and reheat without boiling. Garnish with cayenne pepper and small pieces of lobster. Serve in a soup bowl on a dish decorated with small claws and lemon wedges.

468 calories, 2.1 mg vitamin E, per person.

LOBSTER MAYONNAISE
(*Mayonnaise de Homard*)

1 cooked lobster	sliced cucumber
mayonnaise	tomatoes, red radishes
hard-boiled (hard-cooked) egg	anchovy fillets, capers

Split the lobster down the centre with a sharp knife. Remove
the stomach and intestinal cord (long black line running along
to tail). Twist off the claws, crack, and try to take out the meat
in one piece. Add the meat from the body. Mix with a little
mayonnaise and replace in the shells. Garnish the bottom of a
salad bowl or serving dish with lettuce leaves, and season them
slightly. Lay the lobster upon these, and cover with more
mayonnaise sauce. Garnish with anchovy fillets, capers, hard-
boiled (hard-cooked) egg, radishes, cucumber and tomato.

TO MAKE MAYONNAISE

2.5 ml (½ tsp) salt	2 egg yolks
2.5 ml (½ tsp) dry mustard	150–275 ml (¼–½ pt/
2.5 ml (½ tsp) pepper	½ cup + 2 tbls–1¼ cups) olive oil
	vinegar to taste

Ensure that the eggs and the oil are the same temperature, not
too cold. Remove all traces of egg white from the yolks. Add
pepper, salt and mustard to beaten egg yolks, and drop by drop
add the oil, beating vigorously. If the mixture gets too thick
add a few drops of vinegar or lemon juice. If the mixture should
curdle, break a fresh egg yolk, and beat into this the curdled

mixture. If using an electric blender, put in egg yolks, salt, mustard and pepper. Switch on for a couple of seconds, then pour in the oil slowly.

LOBSTER NEWBURG
(*Homard à la Newburg*)

1 cooked lobster
75 g (3 oz/⅓ cup) butter
75 ml (5 tbls) dry sherry
salt, pepper

150 ml (¼ pt/½ cup + 2 tbls) double (heavy) cream
3 egg yolks, beaten

Cut the lobster in half, crack the claws, remove all meat, and cut into cubes. Season with salt and pepper and cook gently in the butter for a few minutes. Add the sherry, and continue simmering until the liquid is reduced by half. Set a bowl over a saucepan of boiling water and put in egg yolks (broken) and cream, and stir. Do not boil, but cook sufficiently to be of a consistency to coat the back of a wooden spoon. Divide the lobster and liquor equally on to the serving dishes, pour the sauce over it, and sprinkle lightly with cayenne pepper.

928 calories, 4.5 mg vitamin E, per person.

CREAMED LOBSTER

1 small cooked lobster (or
   canned or frozen)
25 g (1 oz/2 tbls) butter
2 egg yolks
60 ml (4 tbls) cream

salt, white pepper
grated nutmeg
3 slices toast, cut into fingers
   or other shapes
chopped (minced) parsley

Split the lobster, crack the claws, and remove all the meat. Cut into thin slices. Heat the butter, and cook the meat slowly in it for five minutes. Mix the egg yolks, cream and seasonings together, and then add to the lobster. Cook very gently until the mixture thickens, but do not boil. Serve on small pieces of toast, and garnish with chopped parsley.

633 calories, 3.5 mg vitamin E, per person.

LOBSTER COCKTAIL

lobster meat (cooked fresh,
   canned or frozen)
shredded lettuce

cocktail sauce (see below)
slices of lemon

Shred the lettuce very finely and place in the bottom of a glass. Do not allow the length of the shreds to be too long. Arrange small lobster pieces on top, and pour sauce over. The sauce may be bought, or your own made to the recipe below, very simply. Garnish with slices of lemon, and small claws if available. Serve as cold as possible.

COCKTAIL SAUCE
(may also be used for prawn/shrimp cocktails)

45 ml (3 tbls) mayonnaise
15 ml (1 tbls) tomato
ketchup (catsup)
15 ml (1 tbls) Worcestershire
sauce

2.5 ml (½ tsp) very finely
chopped (minced) onion
2 drops chilli sauce
pinch celery salt
lemon juice

Mix all the ingredients together, and add lemon juice to taste.

395 calories, 3.2 mg vitamin E, per person.

Mussels (Moules)

Allow 850 ml (1½ pts/3¾ cups or about 2 dozen) of mussels per person. Mussels should be bought whilst still alive, and you should make sure their shells are tightly closed. Throw away any that do not close immediately when given a sharp tap, as they will probably be dead. Also discard any with broken shells.

TO PREPARE

Scrub the mussels with a stiff brush under cold running water, and make sure they are carefully cleaned, removing any sand and grit from inside. Soak for approximately one hour, then drain.

MOULES (MUSSELS) CATALANE

1.7 l (3 pts/7½ cups or about 4 dozen) mussels
150 ml (¼ pt/½ cup + 2 tbls) white wine
1 chopped (minced) onion
sprigs of parsley
lemon juice
150 ml (¼ pt/½ cup + 2 tbls) water
25 g (1 oz/2 tbls) butter
25 g (1 oz/¼ cup) flour
pepper

Scrub the mussels well, discarding any that are broken, and that do not shut when tapped. Place in a large saucepan with water, sprig of parsley, onion and pepper, and heat until the mussels open. Remove the mussels, discard one half of each shell, and cut off the beards. Heat the butter in a saucepan, add the flour, stirring constantly, and cook for a few minutes. Slowly add the wine, keeping the sauce smooth, and then strain the cooking liquor from the mussels into the sauce, heat and beat until smooth. Add lemon juice to taste. Coat the mussels with the sauce and arrange on a dish, garnished with slices of lemon, and sprigs of parsley.

318 calories, 2.17 mg vitamin E, per person.

MUSSELS MARINERS STYLE
(*Moules Marinière*)

This is the most famous of the mussel recipes.

1.7 l (3 pts/7½ cups or about 4 dozen) mussels	25 g (1 oz/2 tbls) butter
1 shallot chopped (minced) finely	150 ml (¼ pt/½ cup + 2 tbls) dry white wine
1 bouquet garni	30 ml (2 tbls) chopped parsley

Melt the butter in a large saucepan over a medium heat. Add the shallots and fry until cooked, but not brown. Add the wine together with the bouquet garni and salt and pepper, and bring to the boil. Boil rapidly for about 3 minutes. Reduce the heat to low. Add the mussels, cover the pan and cook over a high heat until the mussels open. Shake the pan occasionally so that the mussels change places and cook evenly. Discard any mussels that remain closed after 5–10 minutes.

Take out the mussels and discard the empty shell halves. Remove the beards from the mussels and place them in a warmed serving dish. Bring the liquid to the boil for 2 minutes, and then strain it over the mussels. Sprinkle the chopped (minced) parsley over and serve.

257 calories, 2.17 mg vitamin E, per person.

MUSSEL SOUP (*Potage aux Moules*)

575 ml (1 pt/2½ cups or
  about 18) mussels
25 g (1 oz/2 tbls) butter
20 g (¾ oz/3 tbls) flour
575 ml (1 pt/2½ cups) milk
1 bunch parsley

5 ml (1 tsp) white vinegar
150 ml (¼ pt/½ cup + 2
  tbls) white wine
15 ml (1 tbls) chopped
  (minced) parsley
1 egg yolk
30 ml (2 tbls) cream

Scrub the mussels well, and discard any that do not close immediately when tapped. Place in a large pan with the wine, salt, pepper and parsley, and heat slowly until the mussels open. Take out all the mussels and remove the beards. Heat the butter in a saucepan, add the flour, and cook on a low heat for a couple of minutes. Add the milk, a little at a time, stirring constantly, and bring to the boil.

Stir the liquid from the mussels into the sauce, together with the vinegar, and season to taste. Add the mussels, either removed from the shells, or still in them, and heat gently. Mix the egg yolk and cream together, add a little soup to the mixture, and then pour it all into the bulk of the soup and heat to just below boiling point, and then cook a little longer without allowing to boil. Sprinkle chopped (minced) parsley over it and serve.

487 calories, 1.89 mg vitamin E, per person.

Oysters (Huitres)

Oysters are the only shellfish that are eaten raw, and they have the best reputation for digestability and flavour. They used to be both plentiful and cheap in Britain. In fact they used to be classed as the food of the poor! However, in about 1850 they became very scarce, and have remained a luxury ever since. In many places they are in season from autumn to spring only, although they may be bought throughout the year either frozen or canned.

Unless you are expert, do not attempt to open them yourselves — get your fishmonger to do it for you. In shells they are usually sold by the dozen, and must be alive when bought. Shelled oysters are sold by the pint or quart. Canned oysters are sold in a variety of sizes of can.

According to Escoffier, the famous French chef, they are the only hors d'oeuvre (appetizer), apart from caviare, which should appear on the menu of a well-ordered dinner, and he considered English oysters to be the best in the world.

Some people insist that oysters should be swallowed whole, others that they should be chewed to release the flavour.

OYSTERS AU NATUREL
(*Huitres au Naturel*)

12 oysters
paprika or cayenne pepper
4 slices wholemeal (whole grain) bread

25 g (1 oz/2 tbls) butter
lemon to garnish (sliced)

Loosen the oysters with a knife, and replace in the deeper half of the shell, discarding the shallow half. Serve very cold, in their shells, on crushed ice if possible, with paprika or cayenne pepper, slices of lemon, and wholemeal bread and butter. They should be arranged in shallow bowls or soup plates and served as soon after opening as possible, in their own liquor. Some people like a little vinegar with them.

366 calories, 2.6 mg vitamin E, per person.

OYSTERS FLORENTINE
(*Huitres à la Florentine*)

12 oysters	25 g (1 oz/¼ cup) flour
350 g (12 oz) raw spinach leaves	75 g (3 oz/¾ cup) grated cheese
275 ml (½ pt/1¼ cups) milk	seasoning
40 g (1½ oz/3 tbls) butter	

Shred and cook the spinach, and garnish the bottom of the shells with it. Poach the oysters and set one in each shell on the bed of spinach. Coat with cheese sauce, saving some of the cheese to sprinkle on top, and brown lightly under the grill. Serve immediately.

TO MAKE CHEESE SAUCE

Melt the butter in a saucepan, add the flour, and stir with a wooden spoon, on a low heat for 2 or 3 minutes. Add the milk, slowly at first, stirring all the time, until all the milk is in the saucepan. Bring to the boil, add the cheese and cook for a further few minutes, stirring occasionally. If the sauce is lumpy, give it a good whisk.

670 calories, 6.5 mg vitamin E, per person.

STEWED OYSTERS

12 oysters (shelled or canned)   salt, pepper, grated nutmeg
milk   4 slices wholemeal (whole
                                     grain) bread and butter

Poach the oysters in sufficient milk to cover, then season with salt, pepper and nutmeg. Serve immediately with wholemeal (whole grain) bread and butter.

481 calories, 2.8 mg vitamin E, per person.

GRILLED OYSTERS (*Huitres grillées*)

12 oysters   6 slices wholemeal (whole
breadcrumbs   grain) and butter
melted butter

Discard shells and liquor, if using fresh oysters, and roll in breadcrumbs. Flatten in palms of hands, and grill 2 minutes on each side. Brush with melted butter, and serve on hot buttered toast.

646 calories, 3.2 mg vitamin E, per person.

DEVILLED OYSTERS
(Huitres à la Diable)

12 oysters in shells
25 g (1 oz/2 tbls) butter
salt

cayenne pepper
4 slices wholemeal (whole
grain) bread and butter

Open the oysters carefully, loosen the oyster after removing the top shell. Bed the oysters, on their bottom shells, on a bed of kitchen salt on a baking tray. Sprinkle with salt, and plenty of cayenne pepper, and set a small knob of butter on each. Place in a hot oven for about 5 minutes, garnish with sliced lemon, and serve with wholemeal (whole grain) bread and butter.

358 calories, 2.9 mg vitamin E, per person.

FRIED OYSTERS (Huitres Frites)

12 oysters (shelled or canned)
1 egg
deep fat

flour, seasoned with salt and
white pepper
dry, or golden (packaged)
breadcrumbs

Beat the egg, and add a dessertspoon of water to it. Drain the oysters and dry them in a kitchen towel. Roll them in the seasoned flour, then in the egg, and lastly in the breadcrumbs. Fry in deep fat, about 375°F, 190°C, until golden coloured. Drain on kitchen paper, and serve garnished with watercress and sliced lemon.

448 calories, 2.6 mg vitamin E, per person.

GRILLED OYSTERS WITH CHEESE
(*Huitres Grillées au Gratin*)

12 oysters (shelled or canned)
50 g (2 oz/¼ cup) butter

125 ml (4 fl oz/½ cup)
double (heavy) cream
50 g (2 oz) Parmesan or
Cheddar cheese, grated

Place a flame-proof baking dish under a fairly hot grill to heat, and then lightly grease the inside with butter. Set the oysters, without their liquor, on the dish. Spoon some cream on each, and then the grated cheese. Any butter left over should be spooned onto each of the oysters. Cook under the grill (broil) until the cheese has browned, about 5 minutes, and serve immediately.

710 calories, 3.7 mg vitamin E, per person.

HUITRES (OYSTERS) VLADIMIR

12 oysters in shells
25 g (1 oz/2 tbls) butter
25 g (1 oz/¼ cup) flour
250 ml (8 fl oz/1 cup) milk

pinch of salt
browned breadcrumbs
75 g (3 oz) Parmesan or
Cheddar cheese

Poach the oysters and replace in their shells on a bed of salt on a baking tray. Heat the butter, add the flour, stirring constantly, and cook on a low heat for a couple of minutes. Add the milk gradually, stirring all the time, and slowly bring to the boil. Cook for a little longer on a low heat, beating briskly to obtain a smooth sauce. Spoon the sauce over the oysters, sprinkle the brown crumbs over the top, then the grated cheese, and set under a hot grill (broil) until the cheese starts to brown.

594 calories, 3.0 mg vitamin E, per person.

OYSTER SOUFFLÉ (*Huitres Soufflées*)

25 g (1 oz/¼ cup) flour
150 ml (¼ pt/½ cup + 2
   tbls) milk
salt, white pepper
nutmeg

75 g (3 oz/¾ cup) grated
   cheese
25 g (1 oz/2 tbls) butter
3 eggs
4 large oysters

Slightly poach the oysters. Clean the hollow shells, and bed them in salt on a baking tray.

Make the soufflé mixture as follows. Separate the eggs. Melt the butter in a saucepan, and stir in the flour. Cook for a couple of minutes. Slowly add the milk, stirring constantly to maintain a smooth sauce, and bring to the boil. Reduce the heat and stir in the grated cheese, salt, pepper and grated nutmeg. Remove from the heat and allow to cool slightly, then beat the egg yolks in, one by one. Whisk the egg whites until very stiff, and fold in 15 ml (1 tbls) first into the cooled sauce with a metal spoon, before folding in the remainder of the egg white.

Pre-heat the oven to about 375°F, 190°C, Gas Mark 5. Spread a layer of soufflé mixture on each shell, place an oyster on each, and cover with the remainder of the mixture. Heat the base of the baking tray on the top of the cooker, and as soon as the soufflés begin to rise, put the tray in the oven and cook for about 30 minutes, until well set and golden brown. Serve immediately.

557 calories, 3.1 mg vitamin E, per person.

ANGELS ON HORSEBACK
(cocktail appetizers for special occasions)

12 oysters
lemon juice
12 streaky bacon rashers
  (flank bacon slices)
12 cocktail sticks

watercress
cayenne pepper
salt

Open shells and drain the oysters. Dip each oyster in lemon juice, and sprinkle with salt, and liberally with cayenne pepper. Remove the rinds and any white gristle from the bacon, and then stretch each rasher with a knife, by pressing the flat of the blade hard against the bacon, and sliding the knife away from your body. The cutting edge should be towards you. Wrap each oyster in a rasher of bacon, and hold it in place with a cocktail stick. Cook under a hot grill (broil gently) for about 10 minutes, or until the bacon is crisp and golden. Sprinkle with lemon juice, and arrange on a dish, garnished with watercress.

612 calories, 2.5 mg vitamin E, per person.

OYSTERS ROCKEFELLER
(*a famous New Orleans dish*)

12 oysters in shells
275 g (10 oz) cooked spinach
15 ml (1 tbls) chopped (minced) onion
10 ml (2 tsp) chopped (minced) parsley

2 ml (⅓ tsp) salt
2 drops tabasco sauce
50 g (2 oz/¼ cup) butter or margarine
15 g (½ oz) fresh white breadcrumbs

Spread rock salt 1 cm (½ in) deep on a baking tray. Open the oyster shells, drain them, and replace in the deeper half of the shell. Set these shells into the rock salt, on the baking tray. Put the spinach, onion, and parsley through a sieve, or process in an electric blender, add salt and tabasco sauce, and mix well. Cook in butter for a few minutes, add breadcrumbs, and mix again. Divide the mixture into twelve portions, and spread each over an oyster. Bake in a hot oven, 400°F, 200°C, Gas Mark 6, for about 10 minutes. Serve immediately, with a garnish of lemon slices.

404 calories, 5.7 mg vitamin E, per person.

Parsnips

Parsnips used to be much more popular in the olden days, before being overtaken by the potato. They are in season from autumn to spring.

PREPARATION

Scrub the parsnips, then scrape or peel them under cold running water. Leave whole, or cut into halves, quarters or slices. If old, remove the hard centre core. Cook them in a small amount of boiling salted water, until tender — approximately 30 minutes. Season with salt, pepper and melted butter. Sprinkle with chopped parsley.

BAKED PARSNIPS

Cut each parsnip into three or four roughly equal sized pieces. Boil in salted water for 10 minutes. Strain, and dry the parsnips over a low heat. Put into hot dripping in a roasting tin (pan), or around a joint of meat. Baste the parsnips, turning whilst cooking, and cook for 45 minutes to 1 hour, until brown. Garnish with chopped parsley.

MASHED PARSNIPS

Cook them normally, then mash or sieve the parsnips. Add 75 ml (3 fl oz/⅓ cup) of milk and 50 g (2 oz/¼ cup) butter to each 450 g (1 lb) parsnips, and beat until fluffy.

FRENCH FRIED PARSNIPS

Cook in boiling salted water for 10–15 minutes, or until just tender. Cut into chip (French fry) shapes, and fry in hot deep fat until golden brown, approximately 5–7 minutes. Drain on kitchen paper, and sprinkle over 50 g (2 oz/½ cup) of grated cheese to every 450 g (1 lb) parsnips. Serve immediately.

PARSNIP FRITTERS

These may be deep fried or shallow fried.
1) Deep fried — cut the cooked parsnip into chunks, coat in batter, and deep fry until golden brown.
2) Shallow fried — mash the cooked parsnips, season, shape into flat cakes, coat in flour, and fry in butter until golden-coloured.

GLAZED PARSNIPS

Heat 25 g (1 oz/2 tbls) butter, 25 g (1 oz/¼ cup) sugar, and 40 ml (2 tsp) of water in a frying pan (skillet), add the cooked parsnips, and carry on cooking until golden brown.

Peppers

Peppers originated in South America, and may be bought green or red, depending on their ripeness. Choose firm shiny ones. They are at their cheapest from mid-summer to autumn, but like tomatoes may be obtained all the year round.

DEEP-FRIED PEPPER RINGS

Slice the pepper in rings. Beat an egg and coat the slices in this, then in fine breadcrumbs. Deep fry in hot fat, and drain on a kitchen towel.

SHALLOW FRIED

Cut the peppers into strips lengthwise, cover with boiling water and simmer for three minutes. Drain. Fry in hot dripping until golden. Season with salt and pepper.

AS AN HORS D'OEUVRE (APPETIZER) OR WITH A SALAD

Cut pepper in half, remove seeds and white ribs. Drop into hot water for 2 minutes. Chop it finely. Chop a hard-boiled (hard-cooked) egg finely. Mix both together with a little mayonnaise. Season to taste.

PEPPERS AU GRATIN

Prepare peppers in normal manner, and slice thinly. Place on buttered toast. Sprinkle plenty of grated cheese over, and a few small pats of butter. Place under a hot grill (in the broiler) until golden brown.

TO PREPARE FOR STUFFING

Cut off the stem end from the peppers. If they are very large, cut the peppers lengthwise into halves or quarters. Remove the seeds and the inner white ribs. Drop into boiling water, remove from the heat, and leave for 5 minutes. Drain well and stuff with any mixture you fancy. Bake for about 30–35 minutes in a fairly hot oven, 375°F, 190°C, Gas Mark 5.

PEPPERS STUFFED WITH CHEESE AND RICE

2 large peppers
175 g (6 oz/1 cup) cooked rice
50 g (2 oz/½ cup) grated Cheddar
100 g (4 oz) mushrooms (chopped)

75 ml (3 fl oz/6 tbls) single (light) cream
salt and pepper

Cut the tops off the peppers, remove the insides, cover with boiling salted water, leave for 3 minutes. Drain well. Mix the rice, cheese, cream and mushrooms together, and season to taste with salt and pepper. Stand peppers in a buttered baking dish, and fill with the mixture. Cook in the middle of a moderate oven, 350°F, 180°C, Gas Mark 4, for 15–20 minutes.

STUFFED PEPPERS CHINESE STYLE

2 peppers
1 clove garlic, crushed
175 g (6 oz) minced pork

1 spring onion (scallion),
    chopped (minced)
grated rind of ½ lemon
10 ml (2 tsp) oil

Heat the oil in a frying pan, add the garlic and fry until lightly browned. Add the pork and cook for another couple of minutes. Then add the spring onion (scallion) and the lemon rind, and stir for one minute. Take off the heat. Cut the peppers into quarters, remove the seeds and white membranes, and divide the cooked mixture between them. Set these on a greased casserole dish in a medium hot oven 400°F, 200°C, Gas Mark 6, for 25 minutes, or until tender.

Potatoes

Surprisingly, potatoes are a very good source of vitamin C, and not as fattening as is usually imagined. We have already discussed their history, and I do not intend to give recipes for the common boiled, mashed, and roast varieties. The French names for these common methods are given below for your edification and titivation. After all, which sounds sexier on a menu — 'chips' or 'pommes de terre frites à l'Anglaise'?

Boiled potatoes	= Pommes de terre à l'Anglaise
Chips	= Pommes de terre frites à l'Anglaise
Crisps	= Chips
Baked potatoes	= Pommes de terre au four
Roast potatoes	= Pommes de terre château
Creamed potatoes	= Pommes de terre purées

Some other names and brief methods of preparation are as follows.

POMMES DE TERRE À LA BOULANGÈRE

Sliced onions and potatoes fried in butter, seasoned, placed in a baking dish with a little consommé, and cooked in the oven. Proportions: 4 large onions to 8 large potatoes.

POMMES DE TERRE À LA DUCHESSE

Boil the potatoes, drain them and pass them through a sieve. Add butter, and thicken with egg yolks. Usually piped, brushed with egg, and browned. Proportions: 25 g (1 oz/2 tbls) butter and 3 egg yolks to 900 g (2 lb) potatoes.

CROQUETTES DE POMME DE TERRE

Prepare 'duchesse' potatoes as above, roll into small sausage shapes, egg and breadcrumb, then deep fry until golden brown.

POMMES DE TERRE EN ALLUMETTES

Cut potatoes into matchstick sizes, and deep fry.

POMMES DE TERRE SOUFFLÉES

Peel the potatoes, trim square, cut into 3 mm slices, and fry in deep fat until cooked. Remove, and then immerse them in hotter fat, so that they puff up.

GRATIN DE POMMES DE TERRE À LA DAUPHINOISE

Peel the potatoes, cut into slices, place in a buttered baking dish with salt, pepper, grated nutmeg, beaten egg, milk and grated cheese. Mix all the ingredients up, sprinkle more cheese over the top, and cook in a moderate oven for 40–45 minutes. Proportions: 900 g (2 lb) potatoes, 1 egg, 850 ml (1½ pts/3¾ cups) milk, 100 g (4 oz/1 cup) grated cheese.

POMMES DE TERRE À LA HONGROISE

Fry some chopped onion in butter with paprika, add sliced tomatoes, then thick slices of potato, and moisten with stock. Cook until all the liquid has been reduced, and sprinkle with chopped (minced) parsley. Proportions: 100 g (4 oz) onions, 2 tomatoes, 900 g (2 lb) potatoes.

POMMES DE TERRE GRATINÉES

Creamed potato sprinkled with grated cheese, and small pieces of butter, then browned under the grill (in the broiler).

POMMES DE TERRE SAUTÉES

Bake the potatoes in their jackets, peel, cut into slices, place in a frying pan with hot butter and toss until golden.

POMMES DE TERRE À LA LYONNAISE

Toss some sliced onions in butter until golden, and add them to sauté potatoes. Proportions: 900 g (2 lb) potatoes, 225 g (½ lb) onions.

POMMES DE TERRE MACAIRE

Skin some baked potatoes and mash them with a fork, adding seasoning and butter. Form into the shapes of small flat scones (pancakes), and fry in butter. Proportions: 40 g (1½ oz/3 tbls) butter per 450 g (1 lb) potatoes.

POMMES DE TERRE MARQUISE

These are Duchesse potatoes with tomato purée (paste) added. Proportions: 15 ml (1 tbls) tomato purée (paste) per 450 g (1 lb) potatoes, or more to taste.

POMMES DE TERRE À LA MENTHE

New potatoes boiled with a bunch of mint in the water. Garnish each potato with a leaf from the bunch.

POMMES DE TERRE MOUSSELINE

Mashed potatoes with butter, egg yolks and whipped cream added. Usually served in a pastry case. Proportions: 450 g (1 lb) potatoes to 100 g (4 oz/½ cup) butter, 2 egg yolks, 75 ml (4 fl oz/6 tbls) cream.

POMMES DE TERRE PERSILLÉES

Plain boil the potatoes and roll them in melted butter and chopped (minced) parsley.

POMMES DE TERRE SURPRISE

Bake the potatoes in their skins. When cooked, make a small slit, scoop out the potato, mash, season, add cream and butter, and refill the jacket.

Amazing what you can do with a potato, isn't it?

Spinach

Spinach has been cultivated for many centuries, and is an excellent source of vitamins A, C and E, as well as calcium. It is in season all the year round, but is best in the spring. Allow about 225 g (½ lb) per person. Cut off the root ends and wash well, several times if need be. Cook in a saucepan with a tight-fitting lid, with only the water that clings to the leaves, and a little salt, for 10–15 minutes. Stir occasionally. Drain well. To finish, rub through a sieve or chop (mince) finely, and season with salt and pepper. Reheat in butter.

SPINACH ENGLISH STYLE
(*Épinards a l'Anglaise*)

Carefully shred the spinach, boil in the normal manner, drain well, and serve immediately.

144 calories, 9.2 mg vitamin E, per lb.

SPINACH WITH CHEESE
(*Épinards au Gratin*)

450 g (1 lb) spinach   150 g (5 oz/1¼ cups) cheese
75 g (3 oz/6 tbls) butter   salt and pepper

Cook the spinach, drain well, and chop (mince) finely. Melt the butter in a pan, add the spinach and dry it over a high flame. Add half the cheese, seasoning, and cook for a couple of minutes, still stirring. Place this on a buttered flameproof dish, and sprinkle the rest of the cheese over the top. Grill (broil) using high heat until the top is golden.

687 calories, 6.0 mg vitamin E, per person.

SPINACH WITH POACHED EGGS
(*Épinards aux Oeufs Pochés*)

---

450 g (1 lb) spinach   butter
4 poached eggs

Cook the spinach, chop (mince) finely, toss in a little melted butter, and season. Poach the eggs and make each into a neat circle by trimming off any surplus white. Lay these pieces of egg white, chopped roughly, on a heated dish, and cover with the spinach. Flatten the spinach and make four indentations with the back of a spoon. Carefully place the eggs in the hollows, and garnish the outside with triangles of fried bread.

395 calories, 6.68 mg vitamin E, per person.

SPINACH BAKE

450 g (1 lb) spinach
75 g (3 oz/6 tbls) butter
10 ml (2 tsp) chopped
  (minced) parsley

pinch of salt and pepper
3 eggs, lightly beaten
100 g (4 oz/¾ – 1 cup)
  finely grated cheese

Wash the spinach well, and drain. Chop it up, add salt and
chopped parsley, and toss in melted butter. Spread it on a shallow baking tray. Mix the eggs, cheese, and pepper together.
Make two hollows or holes in the spinach, and divide the cheese
mixture between the two. Bake in a medium hot oven, 400°F,
200°C, Gas Mark 6, for 30 minutes.

754 calories, 7.37 mg vitamin E, per person.

SPINACH PANCAKES
(*Crêpes aux Épinards*)

Yorkshire (batter) pudding
  mix (see below)
spinach

50 g (2 oz/¼ cup) butter

Wash the spinach well, shred it finely, and cook it in a saucepan
with the lid on until almost tender. Drain, and dry it by cooking in melted butter. Season, and add an equal amount of Yorkshire pudding paste. Cook the pancakes in a well-buttered
omelette pan.

YORKSHIRE (BATTER) PUDDING MIX

100 g (4 oz/1 cup) plain
  flour
2 eggs

275 ml (½ pt/1¼ cups)
  milk
grated nutmeg
pinch of salt

Sieve the flour and salt into a basin. Make a well in the centre and add the eggs one by one, stirring all the time, working the flour into the middle. Add the milk little by little, until a smooth batter results. Cover and leave to stand for half an hour before using.

655 calories, 6.21 mg vitamin E, per person.

CREAMED SPINACH
(*Épinards à la Crème*)

15 g (½ oz/2 tbls) flour
15 g (½ oz/1 tbls) butter
150 ml (¼ pt/½ cup + 2
  tbls) milk

30 ml (2 tbls) cream
spinach

Cook the spinach, drain well, and chop (mince) finely or push through a sieve. Place in a frying pan with a little butter, and dry over a high heat.

Meanwhile, make the cream sauce as follows. Melt the butter, stir in the flour, and cook for a minute or two, then add the milk, constantly stirring and beating until smooth. Add 15 ml (1 tbls) of cream, and continue cooking until the sauce is very thick. Remove from the heat, and add the second 15 ml

(1 tbls) of cream. Add the cream sauce to the spinach in the proportions of roughly one quarter sauce to spinach, and simmer gently for 10 minutes.

255 calories, 4.96 mg vitamin E, per person.

Tomatoes

Raw tomatoes are an excellent source of vitamins A and C, as well as vitamin E. 450 g (1 lb) of tomatoes would give you 60 per cent of your vitamin A requirements for one day, over twice as much vitamin C as you need, and 5.5 mg of vitamin E.

450 g (1 lb) of tomatoes a day does seem a bit much, but think of it this way — if you ate two tomatoes a day with a combined weight of 175 g (6 oz) you would have 2 mg of vitamin E, 85 per cent of your daily need for vitamin C, and 22 per cent of vitamin A. Isn't it worth a try?

If you have a freezer, I suggest you stack them away in the summer when they are cheap, and then use them in sauces, stews etc. throughout the year. They may even help to stop you catching a cold!

SALADS

Tomatoes may be used to accompany almost all types of foods. They are usually sliced or quartered, or alternatively may be shaped like a lily, as follows. Using a sharp pointed knife, or potato peeler, make zig-zag cuts all the way round the tomato, making sure that the knife penetrates halfway through, then gently pulling the two halves apart.

As a salad, they are usually served in one of the following ways.

1) Tomato salad. Slice the tomatoes thinly. Season. Pour french dressing over them. Garnish with chopped parsley.

2) Tomato and onion.   Boil the onion and then chop (mince) finely. Slice the tomatoes thinly, and arrange on a dish. Sprinkle the onion over the tomato and cover with French dressing. Garnish with chopped (minced) parsley.

BAKED STUFFED TOMATOES
(*Tomates Farcies*)

Choose firm large tomatoes. Cut a slice from the stem end, and remove the seeds and pulp. Discard any hard pieces. Tomatoes may be stuffed with any number of combinations of fillings, and either the lid replaced or the top sprinkled with fried breadcrumbs. Bake in a hot oven for 20 minutes at 400°F, 200°C, Gas Mark 6. Serve hot and garnish with parsley. Here are a few suggested fillings.

COOKED MEATS

Chop or mince (grind) the meat. Add an equal amount of breadcrumbs to the pulp, season, and add sufficient melted butter to bind. Stuff the tomatoes with this mixture.

SHRIMPS OR PRAWNS

Cut into pieces, add a small amount of cream, season and fill the tomatoes.

RICE

Fry some finely chopped (minced) onion, add cooked rice, tomato pulp and seasoning. Fill tomatoes.

BROCCOLI TIPS (GREENS)

Fill the tomatoes with broccoli tips (greens) dipped in melted butter.

CHEESE

Mix equal quantities of grated cheese and breadcrumbs to tomato pulp, with some chopped (minced) parsley, and bind with melted butter.

TUNA STUFFED TOMATOES (*cold*)

6 large tomatoes	salt, pepper
198 g (7 oz) can tuna in oil	1 hard-boiled (hard-cooked)
mayonnaise	egg

Wash the tomatoes, cut off the tops and scoop out the insides. Flake the tuna into a bowl, chop the hard-boiled egg, and add to the fish together with the tomato pulp, mayonnaise and seasoning. Fill the tomatoes, and place lids on top. Serve on rounds of buttered toast, or on a bed of lettuce.

BAKED TOMATOES

Wash the tomatoes, cut in halves, and arrange on a greased fire-proof dish or tray. Season each with salt and pepper and a pinch of caster sugar. Place a small amount of butter on each half tomato, and bake in a medium heat 375°F or Mark 5 for about 15 minutes, or until soft.

GRILLED TOMATOES WITH CHEESE

Wash the tomatoes, halve, and place on a baking tray or grill (broiler) pan. Season with salt and pepper. Mix equal quantities of grated cheese and breadcrumbs, and sprinkle on top. Grill (broil) for about 10 minutes, under a fairly low heat.

TOMATO SOUP

25 g (1 oz/1 thick slice) bacon
½ onion
450 g (1 lb) tomatoes
425 ml (¾ pt/2 cups) chicken stock
salt, pepper
2.5 ml (½ tsp) sugar
1 bay leaf
30 ml (2 tbls) flour
25 g (1 oz/2 tbls) butter
1 small carrot
grated nutmeg
5 ml (1 tsp) lemon juice
30 ml (2 tbls) cream (optional)
chopped (minced) parsley

Dice the bacon, chop (mince) the onion, and the carrot. Melt the butter in a sufficiently large saucepan for the soup, add the bacon, onion and carrot, and cook on a low heat for about 10 minutes. Stir in the flour, and cook for another minute. Add the tomatoes, then stir in the stock (broth), and bring to the boil. Season, add nutmeg and bay leaf, and simmer for about 30 minutes. Push through sieve, reheat and add lemon juice and sugar. Stir in cream before serving, and sprinkle with chopped parsley.

TOMATOES PROVENÇAL
(*Tomates Farcies à la Provençal*)

450 g (1 lb) tomatoes
salt, pepper
5 ml (1 tsp) olive oil
50 g (2 oz) chopped
  (minced) onion
1 small clove garlic
25 g (1 oz/2 tbls) butter

100 g (4 oz/1 cup) fresh
  white breadcrumbs
chopped (minced) parsley
2 anchovy fillets
50 g (2 oz/½ cup) grated
  cheese

Cut the tomatoes in half. Remove the pips and pulp. Place in a flameproof dish or baking tin (pan), season, and cook for a couple of minutes in the oven. Heat the olive oil in a saucepan, add finely-chopped (minced) onion and crushed garlic, and cook gently without browning. Add the butter, then the breadcrumbs, chopped parsley, seasoning and anchovies which have been pushed through a sieve. Mix all together with a wooden spoon, and fill the tomato halves. Sprinkle a mixture of grated cheese and breadcrumbs over the top. Place in a hot oven and cook until the top has browned.

TOMATO OMELETTE

tomato filling (see below)
2 eggs
10 ml (2 tsp) water

pinch salt
pepper
knob of butter

Break the eggs into a mixing bowl, add the water, season, and beat with a fork. Put the butter into an omelette pan and heat until hot. Pour in beaten eggs. After a few seconds, tilt the pan and move the edges of the setting eggs to the centre, with a fork or spatula, and keep stirring gently until the mixture begins to thicken. Cook until the bottom is set and the top is still moist. Add most of the tomato, remove from the heat, fold in half in the pan, and tip out onto a hot plate. If there is any tomato left, place it on top of the omelette, and garnish with parsley.

TOMATO FILLING

Place two or three tomatoes in a saucepan of boiling water. Remove skins, halve, take out the seeds and pulp. Chop the tomato flesh and fry for a few minutes in butter.

Truffles

Truffles are extremely expensive due to the fact that it has not been possible to cultivate them successfully. In the year 1900 there were two thousand tons of truffles available. This has now dropped to one hundred tons a year. At over £100 ($135) per 450 g (1 lb) (about £20 [$27] per 75 g (3 oz) portion) they are possibly the world's most expensive food. The black truffle died out about 50 years ago in Britain. The French use specially-trained dogs nowadays to sniff them out, and even have their own truffle dog trials, which are rather like sheepdog trials. Truffles are used mainly as garnishes or in sauces, or as an hors d'oeuvre, and are available in cans or jars. They should be served very simply, as in the two following examples.

TRUFFLES CRÊME

Peel and cut the truffles into thick slices, season, place in a frying pan (skillet) and pour champagne over them. Set alight, heat and reduce the liquid, add a small amount of cream and butter. Serve immediately.

RÊVES D'AMOUR

Cook the truffles in champagne with a few herbs for 30 minutes or so. Leave to cool for 24 hours in the liquid before serving.

Tuna

Tuna is also called tunny. It is a large fish, and a member of the mackerel family. It is found mainly in the warm waters of the Atlantic, Pacific, and the Mediterranean. The average weight is between 27 and 90 kg (60 and 200 lb), but they can grow to 450 kg (1,000 lb) or more.

TUNA QUICHE

175 g (6 oz) shortcrust pastry (pie crust) for flan case
198 g (7 oz) can tuna in oil
25 g (1 oz) capers
3 eggs
50 g (2 oz/½ cup) Cheddar cheese, grated
25 g (1 oz/2 tbls) butter
1 onion, finely chopped (minced)
125 ml (4 fl oz/½ cup) single (light) cream

Roll out the pastry and line a 200 mm (8 in) flan dish or ring, and bake blind for 10–15 minutes at 400°F, 200°C, Gas Mark 6, until set. Melt the butter in a frying pan, and cook the onions and garlic for about five minutes until soft, but not brown. Stir in the flaked tuna, season and cook on a low heat for about 5 minutes, then remove from the heat.

Mix the eggs, capers, cream, and half the cheese in a bowl, and stir well. Add this mixture to the tuna and make sure it is all well blended, then pour into the flan case and sprinkle the rest of the cheese over. Bake at 375°F, 190°C, Gas Mark 5 for about 35 minutes, until set, and the top is golden brown.

Total calories for quiche 2565.
Total vitamin E for quiche 19.9.
A quarter of the quiche is 642 calories, 5 mg vitamin E.
A third of the quiche is 855 calories, 6.7 mg vitamin E.

TUNA CASSEROLE

198 g (7 oz) can tuna in oil
1 onion, finely chopped
  (minced)
440 g (15½ oz) can
  mushroom soup
50 g (2 oz/½ cup) grated
  cheese
100 g (4 oz/¾ cup) cooked
  rice
30 ml (2 tbls) chopped
  (minced) peppers
198 g (7 oz) can peas,
  drained

Grease a baking dish. Mix all the ingredients together, and turn into the dish. Bake at 400°F, 200°C, Gas Mark 6 for about 20 minutes. Garnish with sprigs of parsley and quarters of tomato.

647 calories, 6.8 mg vitamin E, per person.

TUNA SALAD

198 g (7 oz) can tuna
2 hard-boiled (hard-cooked)
  eggs
4 tomatoes, quartered
1 green pepper, sliced
lettuce
spring onions (scallions), red
  radishes etc.

Cover a plate in rough shredded lettuce, flake the tuna, and place in the centre. Arrange the remaining ingredients around it. Serve with dressing made up of 150 ml (5 fl oz/½ cup + 2 tbls) mayonnaise, 2 drops tabasco sauce, 25 ml (1 fl oz/2 tbls) Worcestershire sauce, or with a salad dressing of your own choice.

409 calories, 10.1 mg vitamin E, per person.

CHOPSTICK TUNA

198 g (7 oz) can of tuna
175 g (6 oz) egg noodles
25 g (1 oz) finely chopped
  (minced) onion
100 g (4 oz) finely chopped
  (minced) celery
25 g (1 oz/¼ cup) flour
45 ml (3 tbls) milk
50 g (2 oz) cashew nuts

85 g (10½ oz) can
  condensed mushroom soup
sprig parsley
25 g (1 oz/2 tbls) butter
227 g (8 oz) mandarin
  oranges

Cook noodles in boiling salted water until tender, and drain. Heat the butter and fry the onion and celery for a couple of minutes. Stir in the flour, cook for 1 minute only before adding the soup and milk. Bring to the boil, stirring continuously, and allow to simmer for 3–4 minutes before adding the tuna in chunks, and the nuts. Stir gently and heat through properly, whilst lining a serving dish with the noodles. Pour the tuna mixture on top, and garnish with a sprig of parsley and mandarin orange segments.

1072 calories, 9.1 mg vitamin E, per person.

Other Foods

GARLIC .

Garlic is available all the year round, and is a member of the onion family. When buying, make sure the bulbs are firm. These consist of a number of curved segments called cloves. Each of these is surrounded by a layer of thin skin, which should be peeled off. The cloves may be added whole or in halves to dishes, or may be crushed with the back of a spoon. A cut garlic clove may be rubbed round the inside of a bowl used for salad or mixing ingredients.

CAPERS

These are the flower buds of the caper bush, found near the Mediterranean, which have been pickled.

BROCCOLI

Broccoli is available all the year round.

LEEKS

Leeks are in season from late summer to late spring.

BRUSSELS SPROUTS

Brussels sprouts are in season from late summer to spring.

SPRING GREENS

These are young cabbages which are sold before the heart has developed. Use as soon as possible, because they wilt very quickly. They are in season from late autumn to spring.

BLACKBERRIES

Blackberries are in season from mid-summer to late autumn, and should be eaten as fresh as possible, because they deteriorate very quickly.

BLACKCURRANTS

Blackcurrants are a very good source of vitamin C, but are seen for sale less frequently than in the past, because whole crops are bought up commercially. In season mid to late summer.

PEACHES

Imported peaches are available from spring to winter, and English hot house varieties from May to October. Eat them whole, and let your imagination run riot!

Sample Menus throughout the Year

LATE WINTER	SPRING	LATE SPRING/ SUMMER
Oysters Florentine	Tuna Salad	Asparagus Salad
Stuffed Peppers (Chinese Style) Hongroise Potatoes Spring Greens	Spinach Bake New Potatoes (Mint) Grilled Tomatoes	Chopstick Tuna Sauté Potatoes Shallow-fried Peppers
Avocado Citrus Salad and Cream	Cheese and Biscuits	Peach
20.8 mg vit. E; 2084 cals.	*20.4 mg vit. E; 1633 cals.*	*18.4 mg vit. E; 1716 cals.*

SUMMER	AUTUMN	EARLY WINTER
Asparagus Soup	Avocado Tuna Cream	Avocado Cream
Lobster Americaine French Fried Potatoes Broccoli (greens)	Mussels Mariners Surprise Potatoes Glazed Parsnips	Tuna Stuffed Tomatoes Creamed Potatoes Lettuce
Blackcurrants and Cream	Blackberries and Cream	Fruit Salad and Cream
14.5 mg vit. E; 1133 cals.	*28.0 mg vit. E; 1637 cals.*	*21.0 mg vit. E; 1575 cals.*

Appendix I

VITAMIN E READY RECKONER (mg)

	25 g/1 oz	50 g/2 oz	75 g/3 oz	100 g/4 oz	150 g/5 oz	175 g/6 oz	200 g/7 oz	225 g/8 oz	250 g/9 oz	275 g/10 oz
Asparagus	0.71	1.42	2.13	2.84	3.55	4.26	4.97	5.68	6.39	7.1
Avocado pears	0.91	1.8	2.7	3.7	4.6	5.5	6.4	7.3	8.2	9.1
Blackberries	0.99	2.0	3.0	4.0	5.0	6.0	7.0	7.9	8.9	9.9
Blackcurrants	0.28	0.6	0.8	1.1	1.4	1.7	2.0	2.2	2.6	2.8
Broccoli	0.31	0.6	0.9	1.2	1.6	1.9	2.2	2.5	2.8	3.1
Brussels sprouts	0.25	0.5	0.8	1.0	1.3	1.5	1.8	2.0	2.3	2.5
Butter	0.57	1.1	1.7	2.3	2.8	3.4	4.0	4.5	5.1	5.7
Carrots	0.14	0.3	0.4	0.6	0.7	0.9	1.0	1.1	1.3	1.4
Caviare	1.82	3.6	5.5	7.3	9.1	10.9	12.7	14.5	16.4	18.2
Cheese	0.23	0.5	0.7	0.9	1.1	1.4	1.6	1.8	2.0	2.3
Cream, double (heavy)	0.34	0.7	1.0	1.4	1.7	2.0	2.4	2.7	3.1	3.4
Cream, single (light)	0.14	0.3	0.4	0.6	0.7	0.9	1.0	1.1	1.3	1.4
Eggs (whole)	0.45	0.9	1.4	1.8	2.3	2.7	3.2	3.6	4.1	4.5
Eggs (whites)	–	–	–	–	–	–	–	–	–	–
Eggs (yolks)	1.31	2.6	3.9	5.2	6.5	7.8	9.1	10.5	11.8	13.1
Flour, white	–	–	–	–	–	–	–	–	–	–
French dressing	1.11	2.2	3.3	4.4	5.5	6.6	7.8	8.9	10.0	11.1
Grapefruit	0.08	0.2	0.3	0.3	0.4	0.5	0.6	0.7	0.8	0.8
Leeks	0.23	0.5	0.7	0.9	1.1	1.4	1.6	1.8	2.0	2.3
Lemons	–	–	–	–	–	–	–	–	–	–
Lobster	0.43	0.9	1.3	1.7	2.1	2.6	3.0	3.4	3.8	4.3

	25 g/1 oz	50 g/2 oz	75 g/3 oz	100 g/4 oz	150 g/5 oz	175 g/6 oz	200 g/7 oz	225 g/8 oz	250 g/9 oz	275 g/10 oz
Mayonnaise	1.39	2.8	4.2	5.6	7.0	8.4	9.7	11.1	12.5	13.9
Milk	0.03	0.1	0.1	0.1	0.1	0.2	0.2	0.2	0.3	0.3
Mushrooms	—	—	—	—	—	—	—	—	—	—
Mushroom soup	—	—	—	—	—	—	—	—	—	—
Mussels	0.34	0.7	1.0	1.4	1.7	2.0	2.4	2.7	3.1	3.4
Olive oil	1.45	2.9	4.3	5.8	7.2	8.7	10.1	11.6	13.0	14.5
Onions	—	—	—	—	—	—	—	—	—	—
Oranges	0.06	0.1	0.2	0.2	0.3	0.3	0.4	0.5	0.5	0.6
Oysters	0.24	0.5	0.7	1.0	1.2	1.4	1.7	1.9	2.2	2.4
Parsley	0.51	1.0	1.5	2.0	2.6	3.1	3.6	4.1	4.6	5.1
Parsnips	0.28	0.6	0.9	1.1	1.4	1.7	2.0	2.3	2.6	2.8
Peaches	—	—	—	—	—	—	—	—	—	—
Peppers	0.23	0.5	0.7	0.9	1.1	1.4	1.6	1.8	2.0	2.3
Potatoes	0.03	0.1	0.1	0.1	0.1	0.2	0.2	0.2	0.3	0.3
Prawns (shrimp)	—	—	—	—	—	—	—	—	—	—
Rice (boiled)	0.03	0.1	0.1	0.1	0.1	0.2	0.2	0.2	0.3	0.3
Sherry	—	—	—	—	—	—	—	—	—	—
Shortcrust pastry (plain pie crust) (raw)	0.34	0.7	1.0	1.4	1.7	2.0	2.4	2.7	3.1	3.4
Spinach	0.57	1.1	1.7	2.3	2.8	3.4	4.0	4.6	5.1	5.7
Spring greens	0.31	0.6	0.9	1.2	1.6	1.9	2.2	2.5	2.8	3.1
Streaky (flank) bacon	0.03	0.1	0.1	0.1	0.2	0.2	0.2	0.3	0.3	0.3
Tomatoes	0.34	0.7	1.0	1.4	1.7	2.1	2.4	2.7	3.1	3.4
Tomato ketchup (catsup)	—	—	—	—	—	—	—	—	—	—
Tomato purée (paste)	1.96	3.9	5.9	7.8	9.8	11.8	13.8	15.7	17.7	19.6
Tuna (canned)	1.79	3.6	5.4	7.2	8.9	10.7	12.5	14.3	16.1	17.9
Watercress	0.28	0.6	0.9	1.1	1.4	1.7	2.0	2.3	2.6	2.8
White bread	—	—	—	—	—	—	—	—	—	—
Wholemeal (whole grain) bread	0.06	0.1	0.2	0.2	0.3	0.3	0.4	0.5	0.5	0.6
White wine	—	—	—	—	—	—	—	—	—	—

Appendix II

CALORIES READY RECKONER

	25 g/1 oz	50 g/2 oz	75 g/3 oz	100 g/4 oz	150 g/5 oz	175 g/6 oz	200 g/7 oz	225 g/8 oz	250 g/9 oz	275 g/10 oz
Asparagus	6	12	18	24	30	36	42	48	54	60
Avocado pears	64	128	192	256	320	384	443	512	576	640
Blackberries	9	18	27	36	45	54	63	72	81	90
Blackcurrants	8	16	24	32	40	48	56	64	72	80
Broccoli	6	12	18	24	30	36	42	48	54	60
Brussels sprouts	6	12	18	24	30	36	42	48	54	60
Butter	210	420	630	840	1050	1260	1470	1680	1890	2100
Carrots	6	12	18	24	30	36	42	48	54	60
Caviare	32	64	96	128	160	192	224	256	288	320
Cheese	120	240	360	480	600	720	840	960	1080	1200
Cream, double (heavy)	127	254	381	508	635	762	889	1016	1143	1270
Cream, single (light)	61	122	183	244	305	366	427	488	549	610
Eggs (whole)	42	84	126	168	210	252	294	336	378	420
Eggs (whites)	11	22	33	44	55	66	77	88	99	110
Eggs (yolk)	97	194	291	388	485	582	679	776	873	970
Flour, white	97	194	291	388	485	582	679	776	873	970
French dressing	187	374	561	748	935	1122	1309	1496	1683	1870
Grapefruit	7	14	21	28	35	42	49	56	63	70
Leeks	7	14	21	28	35	42	49	56	63	70
Lemon	5	10	15	20	25	30	35	40	45	50
Lobster	34	68	102	136	170	204	238	272	306	340

	25 g/1 oz	50 g/2 oz	75 g/3 oz	100 g/4 oz	150 g/5 oz	175 g/6 oz	200 g/7 oz	225 g/8 oz	250 g/9 oz	275 g/10 oz
Mayonnaise	200	400	600	800	1000	1200	1400	1600	1800	2000
Milk	19	38	57	76	95	114	133	152	171	190
Mushrooms	4	8	12	16	20	24	28	32	36	40
Mushroom soup	20	40	60	80	100	120	140	160	180	200
Mussels	19	38	57	76	95	114	133	152	171	190
Olive oil	256	512	768	1024	1280	1536	1792	2048	2304	2560
Onions	7	14	21	28	35	42	49	56	63	70
Oranges	8	16	24	32	40	48	56	64	72	80
Oysters	15	30	45	60	75	90	105	120	135	150
Parsley	6	12	18	24	30	36	42	48	54	60
Parsnips	16	32	48	64	80	96	112	128	144	160
Peaches	9	18	27	36	45	54	63	72	81	90
Peppers	5	10	15	20	25	30	35	40	45	50
Potatoes	23	46	69	92	115	138	161	184	207	230
Prawns (shrimp)	31	62	93	124	155	186	217	248	279	310
Rice (boiled)	35	70	105	140	175	210	245	280	315	350
Sherry	33	66	99	132	165	198	231	264	297	330
Shortcrust pastry (plain pie crust) (raw)	129	258	387	516	645	774	903	1032	1161	1290
Spinach	9	18	27	36	45	54	63	72	81	90
Spring greens	3	6	9	12	15	18	21	24	27	30
Streaky (flank) bacon	120	240	360	480	600	720	840	960	1080	1200
Tomatoes	4	8	12	16	20	24	28	32	36	40
Tomato ketchup	28	56	84	112	140	168	196	224	252	280
Tomato purée	19	38	57	76	95	114	132	152	171	190
Tuna (canned)	83	166	249	332	415	498	581	664	747	830
Watercress	4	8	12	16	20	24	28	32	36	40
White bread	67	134	201	264	335	402	465	528	599	670
Wholemeal (whole grain) bread	63	126	189	252	315	378	441	504	567	630
White wine	19	38	57	76	95	114	132	152	171	190

Index

116